Outsmart Your Pain!

The Essential Guide to Overcoming Pain and Transforming Your Life

Lisa Barr, M.D.

ISBN 13: 978-1-7320011-0-7

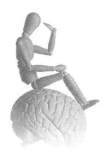

Dedication

This book is dedicated to my beloved family. You are all amazing people who have inspired me to become the best version of me. For this, I am eternally grateful. Your love has motivated me to write this book and work to make a difference in the world.

I also dedicate this book to my patients. Your willingness to allow me to guide you through life's painful experiences is an honor and a privilege. Thank you also to my staff who work diligently to help make magic happen for our patients.

I owe a debt of gratitude to Dr. Alexandria Peck Berger for helping me find my voice as a writer and develop my unique writing style. She is and has been an amazing mentor.

Very special recognition and thanks go out to my father, Gil Binder, for helping me get ready to come forward with my ideas, and for editing the book in its early stages. My appreciation also goes out to Sandi Masori and Mike Koenigs for helping to guide me on this journey. A lot of gratitude goes to my amazing son, Josh Barr, for his patience and expertise in editing this book. I could not have done it without all of you!

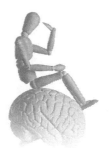

Disclaimer

I want to empower you to overcome your pain and create an amazing life. I wrote this book as a guide that you will hopefully find helpful in your quest to gain mastery over your pain. However, this book is not intended to provide individual medical advice or to contradict the directions and prescriptions of your personal physicians and healthcare professionals.

This book is intended to provide thoughtful information for your consideration. The science of pain is constantly changing. As such, this book is a living expression of where we are now in our overall understanding of pain. This book in no way constitutes the establishment of a doctor-patient relationship. Please seek medical supervision from licensed healthcare professionals before attempting to do anything recommended in this book. Please be careful with your most precious gift: your health.

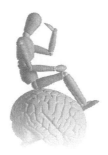

Stay Informed

Please stay informed and updated! I encourage you to visit my website at www.LisaBarrMD.com or connect on my Facebook page at www.facebook.com/LisaBarrMD.

If you want to share your story about overcoming pain or learn how I might be able to help you in my medical practice, I would love to hear from you!

I will be frequently updating this book with new information, patient stories, resources, and helpful tips to help you on your journey to master pain.

To make sure *Outsmart Your Pain* is always updated on your Kindle, go to your Amazon account, scroll to Manage Your Content and Devices, select the Settings tab, and enable Automatic Book Updates.

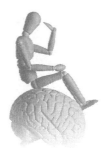

My Promise To You

Dear Readers, thank you for allowing me to accompany you on your healing journey. The purpose of this book, and my mission in life, is to help you gain a better perspective of what pain is, what it isn't, and what you can do about it.

One of the priorities of this book is to help you take charge of your pain and related health issues. Like me, as I will share in the introduction, we all need a little help to feel better from time to time, whether it's through medication, physical therapy, injections, surgery, or other healing modalities.

In other circumstances, our bodies are able to adapt, but we still need to learn how to master mind over matter. Changing your mindset will strengthen your resolve and lead to healing. Understanding how you are affected by stress is also critically important. How we choose to allow painful and traumatic experiences to affect us can either send us into the path of darkness, depression, and disability, or it can positively lift us towards our greatest selves.

I hope that this book will help you to decide what options you have, so that you can become your own best advocate. You have the right to ask questions and speak your mind, especially to the health professionals you consult. If what you're hearing makes no sense or intimidates you, go elsewhere. Rather than giving away your power, use it to enable yourself to make the right choices for you.

Part of my job as a doctor is to teach you to enjoy life's full bounty, experiencing it without fear. I also strive to show you how you can tap into your own inner tools and resources, which have always been there, but may have been previously difficult to access as you struggled with pain and stress.

It has become cliché to say that 'knowledge is power.' But in sharing my insights, which I've garnered treating pain over the many years in medical practice, I hope to help prepare you to bravely face whatever comes your way in life. My promise to you is that I do just that. In turn, I hope you will promise yourself to fully embrace positive change. All it takes is a little curiosity and courage!

"Life shrinks or expands in proportion to one's courage."

- Anais Nin

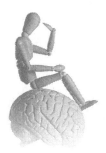

Table of Contents

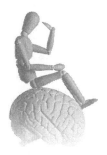

Introduction

"The secret of joy is the mastery of pain."

- Anais Nin

Are you searching for the secrets to mastering pain? Well, I'm glad you're reading my book, because I'm here to help!

Thanks to neuroscience and the growing recognition of mind-body medicine, our understanding of the nature of pain has changed greatly in recent years. Pain is elusive. Many people have a difficult time describing it. We feel it in the physical body, but the pain trigger is often hidden deeper within. We feel pain, but we can't always see or touch it. It defies our senses. It often eludes MRI scans and X-rays. Why? Current science shows us that pain is largely a construct of our minds, and without that influence, we actually don't experience pain. For example, patients with dementia - who previously experienced chronic pain - will eventually stop experiencing symptoms, because they're no longer aware of the pain.

We separate pain into two general categories. Acute pain is present for less than three to six months, and is quite different from chronic pain, which usually lasts longer than six months. Studies confirm that these are entirely different conditions, requiring vastly different approaches. The good news is that, while pain is unavoidable, we have built-in bodily mechanisms designed to reduce or eliminate pain. We just have to learn how to operate the controls.

Importantly, the brain loves information. Since pain occurs in the brain, it's critical to understand the role that learning plays in the new approaches to treatment. That's one of the goals of this book.

In Chapter 1, you'll learn about the different types of pain, and why it sometimes hurts to be human. Then in Chapters 2 through 5, you'll explore how the brain perceives and modulates pain, as well as what happens in the brain and nervous system when things in life are not going well and we're stressed and afraid. In so many words, pain and stress are flip sides of the same coin; the brain and nervous system cannot distinguish between the two. The very same biochemical, hormonal, and immune functions take place in both states. This is what neuroscience is continually demonstrating and proving. This is also what yoga and mindfulness-based stress reduction programs have asserted for decades.

In Chapters 6 through 8, we'll explore how to 'release' and let go of pain, as well as explore various treatment options and ways to improve your habits and achieve wellness. The conclusion of the book will address the transformational aspects of pain and how understanding pain can help you become more self-aware and improve your overall health.

We live in a chaotic world full of challenges that sometimes throw us off-kilter. Our ability to maintain a balance in our lives is the key to health and happiness. But, not all stress is bad for us. Some stress motivates us to focus and perform better. We call this 'eu-stress.' It requires us to consciously make physiological and behavioral changes that balance the effects of our autonomic nervous system, which is the master control center of stress in the body. You'll learn much more about this phenomenon in the first half of the book.

When stress is short-term, and we're able to adapt and cope well with the challenge at hand, we feel excited. This positive mental and emotional state is brought about by the release of 'feel good' chemicals in the brain and nervous system, such as endorphins, oxytocin, serotonin, and dopamine. This positive experience of stress expands our sense of mastery. Being able to adapt, change, and cope with both our internal and external environments is called 'allostasis.' It allows us to find a sense of inner balance, comfort, and calm often referred to as 'homeostasis' or the 'wisdom of the body.'

These optimal states of function help our bodily systems work as a healthy integrated whole. Humming is the word that comes to mind. Our mind and body become synced, and in that state of harmony, we start to hum or vibrate at a certain frequency. This complex process of positive adaptation occurs on all levels, from our tiniest cells to our largest organs to everything in between. It even leads to changes in the brain that allow us to rewire old pain pathways. These positive changes in how the brain works can have tremendous benefits. We are electrical beings with energy coursing constantly through our heart, brain, and nervous system. This synchronization process occurs when the various parts of our electrical system are coherent and working together. Learning how to make this happen consciously is how we 'outsmart our pain.' This specific phenomenon will be fleshed out in Chapter 3.

Unfortunately, when we get sucked into the vortex of work, life, and relationship stressors, we fail to adapt effectively, thus triggering a series of compensatory behaviors that create additional stress. Once this state of imbalance reaches a tipping point, we feel stress in the form of increased muscle tension and pain. This is simply called 'distress.'

However, stressors are not always the result of external situations or events. Thoughts, feelings, desires, and habitual patterns of behavior - as well as compensatory postures and movement patterns - also cause distress. Simple things that we don't often recognize can trigger old pain pathways or grooves in the brain that plunge us into distress. This makes finding and rooting out the pain generator even more challenging. Chapter 4 will address 'Pain as a Habit.'

Functional MRI (fMRI) scans have come a long way in identifying the different parts of the brain that process pain, but there's still no way to recognize these triggers clearly. We still need to piece together what's happening, both in our environments and in our emotional lives, that may be throwing us out of balance, leading to stress, and causing us to feel pain.

Here's the key: stress usually manifests itself in ways that we may not identify as stress. We might experience any number of symptoms, such as tension headache, low back pain, stiff neck, high blood pressure, and more. Unfortunately, there are no 'stress detectors' that we can employ beyond those in our own bodies. As such, it behooves us all to become more aware of how stress affects us.

How we feel is completely unique to each individual. There's really no way to objectively measure one's pain. It's a personal experience that's partly hardwired into us from our past experiences, as my own struggle with chronic pain demonstrates.

It was a beautiful sunny day in May, the time of the year in the South when the weather is warm and balmy. My two young children and I had climbed aboard a friend's 22-foot Sea Ray Bowrider for an afternoon boating trip on Broad Bay in Virginia Beach. As we steamed toward the channel leading to the Chesapeake Bay, without warning, the boat accelerated and suddenly struck a sandbar.

At that exact moment, I was moving from the back of the boat to the bow. Having already experienced momentum going forward on impact, I went airborne like a cannonball. As I was flying through the air, I had the sense to grab onto the cleats at the front of the boat, preventing any tumultuous collision into the water. Instead, I smacked head first onto the hard fiberglass of the bow of the boat, suffering what is called a hyperflexion injury of my neck. The heavy impact forcibly bent my neck down into my chest, causing severe compression of my spine. When the boat came to a stop, and still dazed from the trauma, I looked down into about ten inches of pristine water, the sandy bottom visible below.

Within days of the trauma, the pain in my neck and arm escalated, and I began to experience intense muscle spasms. After a week, I developed a burning sensation on the tops of both hands, with pain radiating down my arms. Every time I lifted something heavy, my left arm would start to shake uncontrollably.

Determined to heal myself, I took it easy, using medication to decrease my traumatized nerve endings, and experimenting with traction and neck exercises. Nothing worked. By the second month, I couldn't walk a straight line or even have an orgasm! I woke up nightly with intense left arm pain. At this point, I sought help. An MRI showed that I had severely herniated the cervical C5-C6 disc in my neck. It was compressing my spinal cord as well as the left C6 nerve. I needed immediate surgery.

Although the surgery initially seemed to go well, as I returned to work three weeks later, the pain persisted. After seeing each of my patients, I would go into my office and lay down on the floor to rest my neck. My staff would walk into my office to check on me, surprised to find me on the floor. After waiting several months, I realized that some of the persistent pain was coming from injured neck ligaments. I sought out treatment with prolotherapy injections. Since I was the only physician doing prolotherapy at that time in my area, I had to travel three hours so that a colleague could treat me. After seven prolotherapy injection sessions, I finally started to feel better. However, I still had left arm pain, weakness, and shaking when I would lift anything heavy. As I started to feel better, I started incorporating low-level pilates and yoga, but I was limited by my left arm dysfunction. I was still miserable.

A second MRI revealed that the disc above and below C5-6 had also herniated and there was a bone spur poking into my left C6 nerve. The MRI also explained why I had developed an unusual condition called Ossification of the Posterior Longitudinal Ligament (OPLL), which can occur after severe spinal trauma. This meant that, as a result of the trauma, the deepest stabilizing ligaments that run up and down the inside of the spinal canal (both in front and behind), had calcified and thickened. These adjacent thickened ligaments, along with the herniated discs, were now causing more spinal cord and nerve compression. I needed additional surgery. My search led me to a second surgeon with expertise in 'minimally invasive spinal surgery.' After this successful second neck surgery, I slowly started to recapture my life again. The process of recovery had taken nearly 10 years!

I also realized that, in order to fully heal and achieve real wellness, I needed to find better balance in my life. To me, that meant not working as much as I had in the past and taking better care of myself - both body and mind. Of course, this is a process that I still work on every day.

I have experienced firsthand the common internal sources of distress resulting from pain, including fear, worries about the future, repetitive thought patterns, and unrealistic expectations we have about ourselves (often referred to as perfectionism). In this book, I'll guide you through an exploration of how and why stress and fear cause pain. You will learn about the different kinds of stress and why they matter. You'll also explore how your mental and emotional responses strongly influence what happens in your body, all the way down to your smallest cells and even your DNA. Then, I'll explain how stressors and traumas, both present and from your past, can repeatedly trigger the nervous system to form pain spirals called 'neural pathways,' which perpetuate pain until you learn to consciously stop them.

The first half of the book reviews how stress and pain can become a habit. It will also explore how some of us, through the process of overidentification with pain, become attached or 'addicted' to it. It becomes the central theme of some people's personal stories. As best selling author and teacher Carolyn Myss describes "your biography becomes your biology."

In the second half of the book, I'll discuss a variety of pain treatments for both acute and chronic pain. Then, I will explore how healthy lifestyle habits, such as sleep and nutrition, can reduce inflammation caused by our nervous system running amok, thereby preventing pain from becoming chronic.

The final chapters are about how pain can be our greatest teacher, prompting us to learn challenging lessons that can only be mastered when we have felt enough pain and suffering that we finally summon the courage to change and seek a more conscious alternative. This process of transforming suffering into something better is a key element of healing. By releasing our attachment to our pain, and letting go of our conditioned responses, pain loses its power over us. It is then we 'outsmart our pain.'

As a board-certified physician, in practice for over 30 years, I have had a lifelong fascination with the human body and mind, and their immense interconnectedness. I have been an athlete most of my life, but my own injury, and subsequent difficulties dealing with it, ignited my curiosity to understand why we hurt and how we can truly heal.

Practicing in the field of medicine called Physiatry (Physical Medicine and Rehabilitation) has helped me to develop a unique perspective about pain and human nature. I continue to learn many lessons about pain from my patients - lessons that will hopefully help many more people heal and thrive.

Following my residency training, I continued to seek a deeper understanding of pain and effective pain treatments. Early in my career, I learned osteopathy, which helped me better understand how the body works on a mechanical level. Then, I studied interventional pain management and acupuncture. I was also introduced to a variety of mind-body therapies along my journey, but the importance of these was reinforced as I experienced from my own recovery from chronic pain. Today, I incorporate these techniques with my patients on a regular basis.

My professional and personal quest continues to this day. In my medical practice, I embrace many different methods, modalities, and techniques including osteopathic manipulation as well as modern interventional pain techniques such as epidural injections, joint and soft tissue injections, radiofrequency ablation, and regenerative medicine, which includes:

- Prolotherapy
- Growth factor injections (signaling proteins)
- PRP (platelet-rich plasma)
- Bone marrow derived stem cells
- Fat grafting

These regenerative therapies have proven to be highly effective in treating early-to-moderate stage degenerative joint disease as well as stubborn tendon and bursa issues. These treatment modalities will be further explored in Chapter 7.

More recently, I have embraced an innovative field of medical study called Functional medicine, which seeks unique solutions to complex medical problems using a 'Systems Biology Approach.' The scientific foundation of this paradigm centers on the dynamic interrelationship of how all of our separate parts connect to the larger whole and how interdependent our organs really are. As an example, many people are unaware that the vast majority of nervous system and immune system function are located in the gut. This is not a new revelation. Hippocrates, the father of modern medicine, asserted nearly 2500 years ago that "all disease starts in the gut." Conventional medicine is slowly coming to recognize this reality, but many doctors have not been adequately trained. A person with immune problems may end up consulting many different medical practitioners, without recognizing that the underlying gut issues must be resolved for healing to occur. Also, the trend of doctors being so specialized makes it challenging to recognize the bigger picture - the interconnectedness of the body. Functional medicine is also important because it takes into account the connections between our mental, emotional, and physical well-being.

In the case of outsmarting pain, I will teach you how the brain affects the body, and in turn, how the body affects the brain, often resulting in the experience of pain. To be healthy and in balance on a physical level, our system must orchestrate a complex matrix all the way down to the microscopic level. This matrix consists of trillions of cells, electrical impulses, molecules, hormones, organs, bones, and tissues. When this integrated process is working well, we can live in a healthy state of balance and be pain-free.

Functional medicine teaches us that disease is not about our broken parts. Instead, it emphasizes that 'the devil is in the details' of our life stories. These details give rich context to our lives and provide critical clues to understanding hidden patterns and triggers that result in stress, pain, and disease. Functional medicine also emphasizes the importance of understanding how our lifestyle and mindset influence our health in dramatic ways, as well as how prioritizing healthy habits is crucial to finding our ideal state of homeostasis.

I have come to believe that the physician's role in treating pain is as a collaborator, a mentor, and a partner for change. We can help facilitate healing by introducing people to new modalities and new ideas of how to live and thrive. By opening your life to possibilities for renewal, free from pain, you'll ultimately learn self-love and acceptance. Liberated from the many stressors that used to plague you, you will be able to cope with the challenges of life, and begin to transform and thrive. It's this process of self-awareness that gives us the power to connect the dots of our stories and our health.

To get the most out of this book, I suggest you keep an open mind about what pain really is. I respectfully challenge you to consider the benefits of changing your habits of thought and movement, be open to emotional self-inquiry, and be willing to practice taking small steps forward on a consistent basis. Armed with this newfound wisdom, you will be able to effectively handle whatever life throws at you.

It is my hope that this book will be a guide to ease you through your struggles, helping you to find balance and inner peace, as you grow into the best, most unshakable, version of you.

> **"Many of us spend our whole lives running from feeling, with the mistaken belief that we cannot bear the pain. But you have already borne the pain. What you have not done is feel all you are beyond that pain."**
>
> - Kahlil Gibran

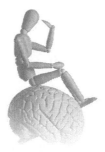

Chapter 1

Pain 101:
'It Sometimes Hurts to Be Human!'

"Our bodies are storytellers. We store memories in our bodies. We store passion and heartache. We store joy and moments of transcendent peace. Our minds may grow numb, but our bodies hold fast to the truth."

- Julia Cameron

Pain affects all of us sooner or later, either directly, or through its impact on friends or loved ones. It sometimes hurts to be human. Hopefully we can all empathize with each other. With our collective power, we can work to make change.

Did you know that more people across the globe are disabled due to chronic pain than any other health condition? Doctors are prescribing more painkillers and performing more surgeries than ever before. As an example, the Centers for Disease Control and Prevention (CDC) reports that opioid overdose epidemic is the fastest growing public health problem in the U.S. The number of people in chronic pain continues to swell. According to researchers from Johns Hopkins University, the annual financial costs of chronic pain now exceeds the combined cost of cancer, heart disease, and diabetes!

Understanding Pain

As you now know, pain and stress have many detrimental effects on the body. To review, pain can:

- Weaken your immune system.
- Impair absorption of nutrients in the gut.
- Make your heart and arteries more vulnerable.
- Decrease your sex hormone production.
- Make you feel pessimistic and irritable.
- Contribute to depression and anxiety.
- Diminish ambition and positive risk-taking.

According to the National Health Interview Survey (NHIS), most American adults report that they suffer from either acute or chronic pain. Approximately 25 million adults experience chronic pain and nearly 40 million adults have severe levels of pain. Additionally, pain-related issues account for about 80 percent of physician visits annually. Consider all of the people in your life affected by the aforementioned symptoms (and many others not listed). The sum total of human suffering is staggering.

This book explores the 'new science of pain,' which has innovative insights that will help us deal with pain more effectively. The following section will explore important foundational concepts about pain that are based on current neuroscience research.

First, pain is an output of the brain, rather than just an input resulting from injury in the body. Pain is actually created in the brain and not in the body.

Second, pain sensitivity and pain intensity can also be solely modulated by the brain.

Third, physical harm does not always result in pain. As such, pain is not an effective barometer of actual tissue damage.

Fourth, pain has an evolutionary purpose. It serves as part of our survival mechanism, protecting us from harm by motivating us to take action.

Fifth, when we feel pain, our brain interprets that pain signal as a threat, causing a stress response that cascades throughout the body. This cascade of systemic electrical and hormonal changes leads to inflammation. Ultimately, if left unchecked, this can contribute to a variety of chronic medical conditions, such as hypertension, heart disease, diabetes, asthma, and more.

Sixth, the brain can get confused, 'thinking' that the body is in danger even when it isn't. This can cause pain when there is no reason. A classic example of this phenomenon is phantom limb pain after an amputation.

Seventh, pain can expand and become a habit. The longer we experience pain, the easier it becomes to feel more of it. The formation of neural pathways or grooves in the brain make it easier to feel pain, which is why we should avoid getting attached to our pain. When we identify with our pain, allowing it to define us, it tends to grow out of proportion, making us feel worse. Pavlov's famous experiments demonstrated that our brain is designed to draw associations between certain activities and experiences. This shows how 'framing effects' work in the brain. In certain contexts, the brain allows pain to be triggered by innocuous stimuli that would usually not cause harm. Examples include social situations, feelings, thoughts, activities, and postures that trigger painful sensations in the body. For example, if you suffer a severe episode of back pain and spasms while bending over to wash your leg in the shower, then you will likely avoid doing this again for fear that you will experience severe pain again. This behavioral response can also lead to anxiety and fear avoidance, which will be explored shortly.

Eighth, pain is tricky because it can be present even when there is no obvious cause. For example, recent research has proved that chronic low back pain can be caused more by social and emotional factors than by the effects of physical tissue damage.

As we proceed through the book, you will learn a lot of scientific information about pain, how it affects the body, and vice versa.

How Our Nervous System Works - The Critical Player

As the critical player in any pain syndrome, it's important to understand how the nervous system works. Our nervous system serves to conduct electrical and chemical messages that transmit energy and information throughout the body. There are four components of the nervous system you will learn about; The Central Nervous System, The Autonomic Nervous System, The Peripheral Nervous System, and The Enteric Nervous System.

The Central Nervous System (CNS) consists of the brain and spinal cord. There are seven distinct parts of the CNS that play different roles in the pain experience. We will explore these shortly.

The Autonomic Nervous System (ANS) consists of the sympathetic nervous system (SNS) and the parasympathetic nervous system (PNS). The ANS is a unique system because it is responsible for coordinating the vast array of automatic activities of the body by releasing hormones and chemicals, that control many bodily functions, such as:

- heart rate
- breathing
- sweating
- secretions of the glands
- blinking
- blood pressure
- overall level of inflammation

These functions operate under the radar of the thinking mind. As you will soon learn, they are theorized to be doing the work of the subconscious mind. The SNS and PNS work as opposites (the yin and yang of the nervous system). Ideally, they work together keeping us in a state of balance called homeostasis.

You will learn in the next chapter that the pair of vagus nerves represent the singular tenth cranial nerve. As the longest nerve in the entire body, it's referred to as the 'wandering nerve,' sending two-way messages from the CNS to all parts of the body, and vice versa. It's central hub or nucleus is located in the part of the brain called the medulla oblongata. It's the common link connecting all four parts of the nervous system into one unified whole. In large measure, it determines our overall state of health and wellbeing because - among other functions - it is responsible for facilitating the body's 'rest and digest' functions.

The Peripheral Nervous System consists of cranial nerves, which stem from the brain, and relate to our senses of sight, hearing, taste, smell, and touch. These nerves also control muscle functions involved in speech and other important areas. Cranial nerves provide crucial information from our environment to the brain. This system also includes spinal nerves that branch out from the spinal cord into the peripheral nerves, which provide electrical impulses to our muscles, allowing us to move at will. The spinal nerves also radiate to our sensory nerves, which actually supply information about our place in the world to the CNS. This creates a two-way street of information going from the brain and spinal cord to our extremities and vice versa.

The Enteric Nervous System (ENS) is one of the main divisions of the autonomic nervous system (ANS), but it's also capable of acting independently. It consists of a mesh-like system of neurons that oversees the function of the entire gastrointestinal tract. Interestingly, the ENS is called the 'second brain,' because it exerts profound influence on everything from gut motility, (which is the transit time of food through our GI system,) to the control of secretions, to the release of acids and enzymes that break down food, so that you can absorb nutrients. The ENS is one of the most complex systems in the body, as it contains more neurons than the entire spinal cord and peripheral nervous system combined.

The role of the ENS in pain is just beginning to be assessed. In my practice alone, we conservatively estimate that at least half of our patients have some sort of imbalance in what we call the 'Gut-Brain-Pain' connection. This can present as reflux, irritable bowel syndrome, leaky gut syndrome, GI infections, malabsorption syndromes, and so on. These issues are in large measure due to the Standard American Diet (SAD), which is rich in highly processed and genetically modified foods, as well as laced with pesticides. No wonder we have so many people suffering from mysterious pain, as well as a variety of GI issues, autoimmune conditions, and psychological issues such as depression, anxiety, and ADD. Our bodies simply don't know how to process and respond to these 'foods' and toxins.

Like many modern Functional Medicine trained physicians, I subscribe to the view that inflammation frequently starts in the gut, even though the effects of the inflammation can be felt anywhere in the body. For example, what appears to be a straightforward knee, elbow, or spinal issue can actually be reflective of a deeper problem, such as inflammation generated in the gut. When this is the case, a more comprehensive approach to treatment is called for, including specialized testing (blood, urine, and stool), as well as the integration of significant dietary and lifestyle changes.

In addition to generating inflammation, the gut can affect our immune function and overall state of mind. When we feel stressed and anxious, we often feel a queasy feeling in the pit of our stomach, or we might belch, feel 'heartburn' or have gassiness. These are just a few of the many GI indicators that our stress response is out of balance. However, many people, including doctors, have not learned about this paradigm. As such, we rarely connect the dots. People end up being prescribed a variety of medications that simply manage symptoms and fail to treat the underlying issues.

In the gut, there are many types of receptors, including those for neurotransmitters that influence our mood, as well as those that modulate our immune reactions. This is an example of why we call the ENS the 'second brain.' This is psychoneuroimmunology at work. Psychoneuroimmunology is a branch of medicine that deals with the influence of our emotional states (such as stress) on our nervous system's activities and on our immune function, especially in relation to the onset and progression of pain and disease. It crosses many different specialties of medicine, and is a scientific basis of many chronic medical conditions as well as of the mind-body connection.

Our gut is also the home of a vast web of bacteria, called the gut microbiome. These are the bacteria that inhabit our intestines and digest our food. Genetically modified and highly processed foods, as well as sugar, are known to negatively affect our gut flora, often wiping out 'good bacteria' and leaving less beneficial bacteria behind. The consequences of an impaired gut microbiome include a myriad of health related issues that masquerade as traditional diagnoses such as reflux, irritable bowel syndrome and ADD, just to mention a few. Our diet, sleep, and stress habits strongly influence our gut microbiome. The effects on the gut microbiome is just one way that lifestyle issues contribute to our overall state of health and ability to overcome pain.

Pain - The Trickster

However, pain is tricky, it's not just a matter of messages transmitted throughout our nervous system. There's so much more to it!

Let's explore one formal generally accepted definition of pain. The International Association for the Study of Pain (IASP) defines pain as "an unpleasant sensory and emotional experience that results in physical suffering or distress that is in response to a real or perceived threat, injury or harm."

I prefer Melanie Thernstrom's definition of pain, as a "complex perception occupying the elusive space spanning sensation, emotion, and cognition." The sensory dimension of pain tells us where it hurts, while the emotional dimension cues us as to how unpleasant the experience is. The cognitive (mental) dimension determines how we interpret the pain based on our past experiences. This multidimensional awareness shows how much deeper the issue of pain can be and how tricky it can be to resolve. We could start by asking ourselves two key questions. Does our pain cause fear and anxiety? How do we respond to the threat posed by the pain?

8

Acute pain is part of our innate survival mechanism, letting us know that we have been hurt or injured. As a purely physical phenomenon, the purpose of acute pain is to warn is of real or potential tissue damage, prompting us to pay attention, and take action if necessary. At this acute stage, pain is usually easy to treat. Think of a broken leg, appendicitis, or a heart attack. When we eliminate the source of tissue damage, the acute pain quickly resolves.

What if You Have Pain All of the Time?

You now know that that pain and tissue damage are not one and the same. Pain can also arise from tension and discomfort caused by our nervous system's response to stressors from external (environmental) factors as well internal ones. Internal stressors include conflicting thoughts, beliefs, emotions, and traumatic or painful memories that quietly trigger our threat response.

I propose that chronic pain arises from a sustained and sometimes intensified threat response mechanism in our nervous system. It behaves like a switch, which gets 'stuck' in the 'on' position. When this switch doesn't shut off appropriately, the influence of the brain and autonomic nervous system (ANS) result in the full systemic effects of chronic pain.

Chronic pain is a complex process resulting in pain that persists when it shouldn't necessarily. This is a function of the brain's internal processor, which can magnify or minimize our pain. The brain's ability to intensify pain is called 'central sensitization.' This is a different kind of warning sign that informs us that something larger is happening under the surface that requires our attention. When pain becomes chronic, symptom-based treatments have limited effect. This is when we need to employ a broader perspective, such as 'The Pain Release Process,' which will be explored in Chapter 6.

9

A variety of predisposing factors have been identified in people who are prone to developing chronic pain. Risk factors can include gender, genetics, psychosocial issues, socio-economic struggles, prior surgical trauma, scars, nerve damage, inflammatory responses, toxicity, infections, autoimmunity, and more. Genetic risk factors have recently been identified in people who are more susceptible to centrally-mediated pain syndromes. Interestingly, these same genes impact the production of the chemical neurotransmitters in the brain that control our pain threshold and impact our mood. These genetic variants are often seen in Fibromyalgia Syndrome (FMS) which is a form of chronic widespread soft tissue pain accompanied by chronic fatigue, sleep disorders, as well as mood and memory changes. Researchers believe that FMS is a form of central sensitization and that it may result from the way your brain processes pain signals.

Based on the contributions of modern neuroscience, we are aware that pain is not purely a physical musculoskeletal issue. For example, functional MRI (fMRI) studies show that chronic pain conditions, such as advanced degenerative osteoarthritis of the hip, can actually lead to physical changes in the brain. The result can lead to the loss of gray matter in multiple areas of the brain, including the amygdala (which stores memories), the sensory cortex (which controls our perception of the world and of ourselves), the cerebellum (which controls movement), and the prefrontal cortex (which controls movement planning and abstract reasoning). These changes in our brain leave imprints or scars. Because of the benefits of neuroplasticity, resolution of pain by definitive treatment, such as a hip replacement followed by proper rehabilitation and gait training, can completely reverse these changes. Neuroplasticity will be the topic of exploration in Chapter 3.

This example illustrates the bi-directionality of our neurological wiring system, demonstrating how the brain impacts pain and how pain is influenced by the brain. This is the two-way street of communication on cellular, molecular, and electrical levels, which stretches between our brain, musculoskeletal, organ systems, and more. Remember that the very same process that results in pain or 'dis-stress,' also occurs when we're stressed.

The root of pain can be physical, mental, emotional, and attributed to stress from traumatic experiences, or any combination thereof. Each person feels and responds to pain in totally unique ways. With this foundational knowledge, we can better understand the brain and nervous system's role in pain. We know that the brain is a complex, three-pound convoluted mass of neurons sitting at the top of our nervous system. But, what about the mind's role?

When Mind Matters

While it's not easy to define the concept of the 'mind,' we seem to intuitively know when we're in our right mind and when we're not. Dr. Daniel Siegel, a psychiatry professor at UCLA, coined the term 'mindsight' to describe the workings of the mind. Some people might like to substitute 'insight,' but he asserts that mindsight is what our mind sees.

He explains that mindsight is "a powerful lens through which we can understand our inner lives with more clarity, integrate the functions of the brain, and enhance our relationships with others. It is a kind of focused attention that allows us to see the internal workings of our own minds, helping us get out of the autopilot mode of ingrained behaviors and habitual responses. It lets us name and tame the emotions we experience, rather than being constantly overwhelmed by them."

Dr. Siegel reiterates that we each have a unique perspective of the world. Not only do we have individual thoughts, feelings, perceptions, beliefs, and memories, we have unique self-regulatory patterns that shape the flow of energy and information inside us. These concepts are extremely powerful in learning to manage the effects of stress effectively so that we don't become distressed and suffer in pain. You'll learn more about this in Chapter 6 when you discover the 'Pain Release Process.'

Now that we have a clear picture of the brain and how it differs from the mind, we need to explore the three levels of consciousness that are functions of the mind. These include the conscious, subconscious, and superconscious minds. For the purposes of this book, I suggest you think of the unconscious and subconscious mind as interchangeable. For the sake of clarity, I will refer to both collectively as the subconscious mind going forward.

First, our conscious mind is similar to a computer processor, capable of retrieving programs, data, and processes necessary to operate our body. The subconscious mind on the other hand is the reservoir of our feelings, thoughts, urges, and memories that are outside of our conscious awareness. It is like the disk storage on a computer. The subconscious mind also serves as the master of our autonomic nervous system, providing balanced functions that protect the body. It facilitates the opposing actions of the sympathetic nervous system (SNS), prompting the fight-or-flight response that keeps us out of harm's way, and managing our automatic functions of rest, digestion, and repair, which are mediated through the actions of the parasympathetic nervous system (PNS).

The conscious mind is the gatekeeper of the subconscious mind, which is much like a small child. It needs very clear and deliberate directions. However, the subconscious mind is also quick to make associations and it takes everything literally, so we must be careful of our words. If you declare 'my boss is a pain in the neck,' your subconscious mind might figure out a way to make sure your neck hurts at work.

No impression enters the subconscious mind that isn't first allowed in by the conscious mind. This is why negative thoughts and conditioned beliefs easily take root and have a harmful impact on our health. This is especially true if we aren't aware of the effect these thoughts have on our subconscious mind and autonomic nervous system. One effective strategy in reducing the unwanted effects of negative thoughts and beliefs is called 'mental pivoting.' I liken it to a mental version of the 'Hokey Pokey' in that it allows you to consciously change the direction of your thoughts and deliberately choose a thought that is positively aligned to your desired health goals.

Our subconscious mind also helps us learn lessons from our past experiences and communicates to us through symbolic language as well as through our emotions. Knowing this can help provide clues about the roots of pain, especially when the cause is not so obvious. Here's an example of pain/body symbolism. Imagine a person with chronic foot pain. They deny a history of significant trauma. They seek treatment, without success. At a certain point, the patient and medical professional become frustrated. The experience of foot pain persists, but there is no obvious tissue damage. When the source of pain is not obvious, it is possible that the subconscious mind may be communicating hidden mental and emotional messages through symbolic body language.

To better understand this, you could 'play with the language' of the symptoms, remembering how the subconscious mind works. You could open a dialogue around what the pain might symbolize. Symbolic pain language is like a puzzle. In this case, chronic foot pain might represent a lack of 'under-standing.' In other words, his feet metaphorically are 'under his standing.' In this case, it might be helpful to consider what is he not seeing clearly or appreciating in his life. When we contemplate both the symbolism and metaphors for our pain, as well as the physical aspects, we can solve complex pain issues more quickly. Pain symbolism will be further explored in Chapter 9.

The Language of Pain

Have you ever noticed that pain can be difficult to describe? Most patients come in to see me with pain, but when I ask them to describe it, they have to stop and think about it. In their silence, I start asking them some leading questions about how their pain feels. Is it burning, sharp, dull, or achy? Where does it hurt? Where does the pain radiate to? I also want to know what makes it better and what makes it worse? When did it start and what may have triggered it?

I have learned that if I listen long enough to a patient's story and their concerns and then ask the right questions, they will eventually tell me what's wrong with them. Because languaging pain is challenging for many people, I also ask my patients to draw their pain on a diagram. I pay close attention to how each person draws and describes their symptoms. Words and images are helpful clues about how that patient sees the world.

The adage is true that 'words have power,' and we need to choose them wisely. Positive words can help you while negative words can harm you. I encourage you to be careful what you say out loud about yourself, because your subconscious mind doesn't miss out on anything. 'Unconscious reactions' to our circumstances perpetuate the negative stories that we tell about ourselves. Examples include people who say 'my pain is terrible and unrelenting' or 'I cannot stop taking my pain medication because I have nothing else to fall back on for relief.' or 'I need medication to function.' Remember that your subconscious mind will accept whatever you tell it. As such, you can expect to experience more of the same , be it good or bad. Practicing the mental pivot is especially helpful when you are hurting and feeling stuck.

Words spoken consciously, with attention and feeling help the subconscious mind spring into action. An example would be, 'I am blessed to have the best medical help and support that I need to overcome my challenges.' In this case, your subconscious mind will not only 'bring you' optimal opportunities for healing, but also encourage you to take advantage of them. By consciously choosing and repeating positive thoughts and phrases about your body, you can trigger positive changes in your health. Knowing how your mind works is critical to your health and your well-being. This is how prayer and affirmations work. This is how you are wired.

You're now beginning to see an expanded view of the mind-body connection. Throughout this book, you will learn more about the intricate web of the mind, emotions, the brain, and the autonomic nervous system, as well as how these connections influence your experience of reality. By mastering these insights, you will be able to take the necessary steps to reduce your pain and suffering and become more vibrantly healthy and resilient for life.

A Historical Perspective of the Subconscious

According to renowned psychiatrists Carl Jung and Sigmund Freud, our subconscious mind influences our behavior and experiences, even though we aren't aware of these influences. Jung famously said that "until you make the subconscious conscious, it will direct your life, and you will call it fate." To resolve issues, one must relinquish the 'secrets' held in the subconscious mind, bring them to the fore, and speak them out loud if necessary to release them from 'bondage.' These are the issues we often stuff in our tissues, particularly in our soft tissues (muscle and fascia). Once these issues have less power over us, and we no longer have to feel the emotional pain and baggage that accompanied them, we begin to feel better.

Paraphrasing theologian E. Stanley Jones, the conscious mind determines our actions and the subconscious mind determines our reactions; and our reactions are just as important as our actions. It's not surprising that humans are so instinctive, because our subconscious mind is more prominent than our conscious mind. With its physical seat in the lower brain (brain stem), the subconscious mind comprises 50 to 60 percent of our brain's total capacity and operates entirely under the radar of our conscious mind. Mastering the 'secrets' of your subconscious mind will help you more easily outsmart your pain. The subconscious mind has many roots bridging the mind and body, including the nervous system, endocrine (hormone) system, immune system, physical body, as well as a connection called the superconscious mind.

While our conscious and subconscious mind are closely aligned with our physical body, our superconscious mind transcends the physical. Our limited conscious mind or 'thinking mind' sees all things as separate, while our superconscious sees everything as unified. The superconscious mind is omniscient and all-knowing. It is the part of our mind that transcends the personal, seeing beyond material reality and gaining access to what Jung described as the 'universal unconscious' (also called the mind belt or zeitgeist).

The superconscious is considered the source of genius, creativity, insights, and novel ideas. Intuition and déja vu experiences are elements of the superconscious as well. The superconscious mind is significant because, like our DNA, it holds the blueprint for what is possible for each of us. Some religious and spiritual traditions consider the superconscious as our Spirit or that part of us that is made in the image of God. Some even refer to it as Christ consciousness.

Our superconscious mind communicates to us by whispering or sending us messages from the 'small voice within,' helping to guide us toward health and our best path forward in life. This 'voice' facilitates synchronicities, which are like signposts pointing us in the right direction. Our superconscious mind can help us identify the course corrections that we need to make in our lives.

Some would argue that pain is a sign that we may not be listening to these internal messages, leading some to self-sabotage. When we are on 'autopilot', and not paying attention to the whispers of the higher self, we might not be consciously aware that our life path is misaligned with our higher purpose. When we get off track, one of two things can happen. The 'universe' can nudge us gently or 'whack us upside the head,' indicating that we need to make a change. Listening to the wisdom of the body and being open to change has the power to free us from the harshest effects of these messages. But sometimes pain is the message we need to do just that.

Pain and the Disease of Denial

Some people subconsciously make pain a habit. Others choose to avoid dealing with painful experiences altogether, retreating into denial mode, and subconsciously choosing to not embody or fully feel the painful triggers. This phenomenon is the subconscious psychological process called 'dissociation of pain.'

At times, our coping strategies are unable to handle the stress of pain. We may compartmentalize the pain in our minds. While this may seem like a constructive coping strategy, it actually makes pain more difficult to assess and treat effectively using traditional means. Rooting out the real underlying issue becomes murky, because the real culprit is often hidden in our deepest subconscious thoughts, emotions, beliefs, and feelings.

Allowing thoughts to flow through our minds without judgment or resistance helps us feel good and generally makes life easier. On the other hand, when we resist and judge our thoughts, those negative or unwanted thoughts get magnified, causing our body to feel stuck. For those who worry incessantly, this phenomenon can have a dramatic effect on wellbeing. Remember that, like our words, our thoughts are proven to have great power, even so much as to alter our body's internal processes. In fact, our thoughts, emotions and words can even alter the expression of certain genes and change the shape of the water molecules that make up at least 60 percent of the body. You'll learn more about this later in the book. For now, you have a greater understanding of the dramatic improvement in overall health that can be achieved if we believe it can happen.

Thoughts and feelings that are repressed, but not forgotten, are stored in our subconscious mind. They tend to play out in our tissues, especially our soft tissues - muscles, fascia, and tendons - through the influence of the autonomic nervous system. In cases of this nature, tens of billions of healthcare dollars are spent trying to put a spotlight on the actual pain generator, as well as help identify unique pain triggers.

However, as long as the core mental and emotional issues remain deeply buried in our subconscious, pain becomes difficult to resolve. These sorts of issues can't be seen on any MRI or CT scan. Unfortunately, doctors continue to order endless diagnostic tests, hoping that a 'smoking gun' will appear. This perpetuates a challenging process of medical hide-and-seek. It also accounts for a large part of our healthcare crisis, both in terms of dollars, but more importantly, in human suffering.

Begin to Outsmart Your Pain

Statistics about the worldwide incidence and cost of chronic pain are staggering and the opioid epidemic continues to harm countless communities and millions of people. According to New York Magazine, the United States "pioneered modern life and now epic numbers of Americans are killing themselves with opioids to escape it." CBS News reported in June 2017 that drug overdose is now the leading cause of death among Americans under the age of 50. According to the New York Times and The Washington Post, life expectancy for both men and women have declined in the last two consecutive years, which is largely attributable to the opioid crisis. Did you know that more Americans die from overdose deaths than died from AIDS at the peak of the epidemic in the 1980s?

One of the factors that contributed to this crisis has been the medical community's emphasis on pain as a 'vital sign.' However, after 15 years, the American Medical Association (AMA) finally changed its stance and no longer promotes pain as the fifth vital sign, realizing a bit too late that their perspective on pain was mistaken.

Pain is unlike the other vital signs (pulse, blood pressure, temperature, and respiration rate) because it is subjective. You may recall your doctor asking you to rate your pain on a scale from one to ten or identify one of a series of illustrated emotive human faces. Since no two people experience pain in the exact same way, there is simply no objective way to measure it. Even neuroscientists, using the latest functional MRI (fMRI) scans and sophisticated computer models, can't measure pain. As science writer Erik Vance asserts, it's shocking that "there is still no way to measure pain beyond asking the person how much it hurts."

Pain is a significant feature of many diseases and conditions. Thus, pain does not 'belong' to any one specialty. There are three generally recognized types of pain. Nociceptive pain stems from muscles, joints, bones, and tendons. Neuropathic pain has its origin in the nerves. Central pain is generated, modulated, or amplified by the central nervous system. All three types of pain require a different treatment approach.

Nociceptive pain would result from a broken bone, arthritis. or tendonitis. The treatment might involve topical or oral anti-inflammatories, mild pain relievers, rest, and possibly a period of immobilization. Additionally, physical therapy as well as ice and heat can be helpful managing this type of pain.

Neuropathic pain has a nerve origin. This could be due to a pinched nerve from a herniated disc in your spine or nerve compression such as carpal tunnel syndrome. Peripheral neuropathy is also a form of neuropathic pain. Cortisone injections can sometimes be helpful for nerve irritation or compression. When that is not appropriate, there are specific drugs that influence neuropathic pain such as Gabapentin, Lyrica as well as various antidepressants and anti-seizure drugs that modulate pain by affecting the nerves and the brain.

Central pain syndrome is much more complex and difficult to treat. This type of pain is believed to be the result of a sensitized nervous system, meaning that the brain and spinal cord amplify pain. Fibromyalgia, which is associated with widespread soft tissue pain, fatigue, mood alterations, and sleep disorders, is a classic example of this phenomenon. Chronic regional pain syndrome

(CRPS) of which there are two types are also believed to be central pain syndromes. These uncommon syndromes can occur after nerve injury, trauma, surgery, stroke, and heart attack. They present unique diagnostic and therapeutic challenges.

Identifying the type of pain you may have will have significant bearing on how best to treat it. Treatment options for a variety of common painful conditions will be further explored in Chapter 7 - The Pain Treatment Toolbox.

Pain Misperceptions

Misconceptions about pain long predate the medical establishment. Since Aristotle and the ancient Greeks, pain has meant many things to different people. It has been relegated to the realms of the heart, believed to be punishment from the 'gods,' blamed on malfunction of the nerves, and ultimately attributed to the brain. In addition, there are vast cultural differences around the idea of pain and how it is perceived. Because pain defies our senses, there's no uniform language to describe how we experience it. This makes optimal communication between the doctor and patient, as well as between the patient and their support system, more challenging.

Neuroscience has shown that the perception of pain is anything but black and white. It's a contextual experience that's highly processed by the entire nervous system, which includes the brain, spinal cord, as well as the peripheral, autonomic, and enteric nervous systems. This network of neural tissue forms the mainframe computer of pain in the body.

We know that the way we perceive and interpret pain is highly dependent on the unique set of circumstances occurring at the time that we first feel the pain. The brain and subconscious mind quickly draw associations about the pain by interpreting external

21

environmental and internal circumstantial clues via input from the senses. This is why no two people feel the same pain in the same way.

Through the formation of neural pathways or 'neural grooves' in the central nervous system, chronic pain can even become habitual, keeping unresolved physical and emotional issues literally stuck in our tissues. Because the brain is 'soft-wired' rather than 'hardwired,' whenever we learn something new, our neural connections change. This is one of the benefits of neuroplasticity, which will be further discussed in Chapter 3.

Dr. John Sarno and the Evolution of Mind-Body Medicine

Research increasingly bears out the validity of the theories of one of my early mentors, the pioneering physiatrist Dr. John Sarno. He was one of the first to write about the complexities of the mind-body connection, calling effects of these stuck emotions 'tension myoneural syndrome' (TMS). Sarno had firm beliefs about pain and how to treat it. He typically prescribed 'education' and physical activity. His approach was to avoid pills, physical therapy, and injections as he felt that these treatments served to reinforce the physical aspect of the pain, making it harder for patients to outsmart their pain. He discouraged his patients from bed rest and challenged them to keep moving, even though they hurt. He emphasized the importance of not succumbing to the paralyzing fear that if we move, our pain might escalate out of control. This is what we now refer to as 'fear avoidance,' the irrational fear of a pain spiraling out of control, which can stop us in our tracks and make meaningful recovery nearly impossible.

Sarno explained that the brain manifests pain as a distraction, so that we don't have to process or feel our uncomfortable and repressed emotions, especially fear, anger, and rage. To overcome this phenomenon, he taught straightforward mind-over-matter strategies that are similar to what is now called cognitive-behavioral therapy (CBT).

To his credit, he predicted the current opioid crisis as far back as the 1980s. This was a time when few people outside of chronic pain sufferers took him seriously. Sarno was also one of the first to popularize the Biopsychosocial Model, which takes into account the intricate interactions of biological, psychological, and social factors on one's health. This is similar to the Systems Biology approach which is the basis of Functional Medicine. Like many pioneers, Sarno held firm to his beliefs and convictions, making his books a treasure trove of insight.

If we are to accept the wisdom of Sarno, Jung, and Freud, we can conclude that repressed emotions often stem from conflicting ideas about what we want and need, and what we think we deserve. Because many of us are fearful about dealing with the pain associated with these internal conflicts, we tuck them away in the deepest recesses of our subconscious mind. We are wired in such a way that when these inner conflicts are not consciously processed and released, they often manifest as physical complaints.

The basic laws of physics apply to humans too. We know that energy can neither be created nor destroyed; it can only be transformed. Thus, the energy of these repressed emotions gets stuck, manifesting itself in physical form as muscle tension, abnormal posture, muscle guarding, painful gait deviations, and even what we dub as 'pinched nerves.'

Dr. Sarno had many revolutionary theories about pain. However, his approach left little room for the idea that sometimes people need a little outside help getting pain relief, so that they can avoid moving into a state of fear and 'overwhelm.'

Humans usually perceive pain as stressful. The brain naturally perceives it as a threat, causing a massive series of changes that are triggered in many of our bodily systems including our nervous, cardiopulmonary, hormonal, immune, and gastrointestinal systems. This process results in a domino effect of cellular and physiologic changes that not only create inflammation and reinforce the pain, but also intensify other medical issues. This is believed to be one of the mechanisms behind central pain syndromes like Fibromyalgia, Chronic Fatigue Syndrome, and Complex Regional Pain Syndrome (CRPS).

The systemic tidal wave of physiologic changes triggered by pain is collectively referred to as our 'psychoneuroimmunology.' This concept of how our mind and body are connected through our electrochemical processes was discovered over 2000 years ago by Hippocrates, the father of medicine, and is one of the secrets of the great spiritual masters. Learning how to consciously control these processes will help to set you free of pain and suffering, while also aiding in the prevention of many other chronic medical conditions.

Unlike Dr. Sarno, I believe in alleviating pain using appropriate treatments, such as hands-on techniques, physical therapy, injections, and even the judicious use of medication, as long as they are just a short bridge to the other side of pain. In other words, the treatment serves as an important step in calming the nervous system and preventing the threat response from being triggered. Appropriately treating pain helps to buy time for healing to occur, allowing people in pain to have a reprieve and a sigh of relief. People can then make mental pivots in the direction of healthier habits. From a place of feeling better, they become more open and trusting and then they can start to learn effective ways to modulate their stress hormones and neurotransmitters. In my experience, when people are suffering to a significant level, it is challenging to simply suggest they just breathe and relax.

I have come to believe that pain is a growth opportunity, teaching us that we can master it by learning to master ourselves. This book is designed to provide you with an introduction of how our system is wired (both mind and body), as well as provide you with some helpful tools that will empower you to live a life beyond pain and suffering.

Time for Change

The effects of chronic pain and stress take place on a spectrum ranging from temporary symptoms to end-stage tissue changes, fatigue, and physical exhaustion. The earlier the intervention to make changes, the easier it is to resolve the condition. However, when treatment is delayed to the point that the body is so far out of balance, the pain will be much more difficult to treat, and the prognosis will change. This is because we all have a certain amount of 'reserve function,' be it cognitive (brain) or physical (body). Learning the early warning signs that our body's systems are out of balance is crucial. This will allow us to avoid crossing the 'point of no return.'

In doing so, we can calm the brain's interpretation of events and mitigate the threat response mechanism. As we begin to feel safe, we can start to approach our deepest issues from a less fearful position. The secret is that we must recognize that the hands-on treatments, injections, or medications are just a starting point, rather than the lasting solution. Helping people feel better facilitates buy-in, building the trust that's necessary to keep the threat response low. Then, people in pain may be more willing to start searching for the deeper triggers and begin thinking about their pain differently.

25

Most chronic pain and many chronic medical conditions, including addictions, can be caused by repressed emotions that have important hidden drivers. Studies show that we are more susceptible to chronic pain and addiction when we lack genuine emotional connections with others and with ourselves. Without a genuine sense of self, and without a meaningful sense of belonging, we can be catapulted into loneliness, isolation, and despair, which can trigger an existential crisis that often manifests as severe pain and addiction.

These kinds of 'felt' conditions certainly cannot be seen on X-rays or other imaging studies. Because of our common humanity, and the vast impact of shame, guilt, and denial, we often don't go to our doctor's offices with such complaints. We are preoccupied, thinking that our pain is caused by a bulging disc, plantar fasciitis, or tendonitis.

One of my goals in writing this book is to explain why the medical community must expand the pain paradigm to be more inclusive of how we assess and treat the many facets of pain. From the failed concept of pain as the fifth vital sign, to the urgent call in the last two decades to not under-treat pain, our healthcare system has thoroughly demonstrated that it often has poor solutions for addressing the pain pandemic. Unfortunately, this is true not just in the United States, but appears to be nearly universal, as similar issues spring up in many countries across the globe.

The old model of assessing pain purely as a symptom is slowly shifting. We are starting to identify pain as the sum total of a myriad of physical, emotional, mental, and post-traumatic inputs. Within this larger, more inclusive paradigm of mind-body medicine, we now know that pain is a more complex and pervasive condition than previously believed. Whether we realize it or not, our thoughts, beliefs, and emotions play a significant role in whether we perceive pain as our friend or foe. This distinction largely determines the rest of the story.

Before we move on to explore the 'Brain on Pain' and the stress-response mechanism, let's review some common myths and truths about pain.

The myths (untruths) about pain include:

- As we age, we're supposed to become less active and it's normal to have aches and pains.
- We can injure ourselves further if we exercise when we're in pain.
- If the doctor can't find the 'smoking gun,' then the pain must be in your head. Maybe it's all in your head!
- All people who take opioids become tolerant and addicted, thus requiring escalating doses over time.
- By ignoring your pain, it will go away.
- We should just push through the pain to get better.
- When we suffer for so long, with many unsuccessful treatments and doctor visits, we'll just have to learn to live with the pain.
- You will always have pain, whether it's from a bulging disc, spinal stenosis, or any other condition.

The truths about pain include:

- Acute and chronic pain are very different conditions. They require different treatment approaches, because the source of most chronic pain is in the brain and nervous system (software), rather than in the painful tissue (hardware).

- Physical injuries can heal, but pain can persist due to faulty movement patterns that develop as a way of compensating for the pain.
- Overthinking your pain, also called catastrophizing, will make your pain much worse. This is quite common and leads to the dissociation of the mind and body.
- Fear and avoidance of movement will significantly delay recovery by maintaining the threat response mechanism in the 'on' position, making it hard to think straight or take effective action to heal.
- Certain personality characteristics, such as perfectionism, make us prone to chronic/recurrent pain.
- Pain signals are a two-way street. 'Downstream issues' in the gut can cause 'upstream effects' in the brain, resulting in pain that can be felt anywhere in the body. I call this the 'Gut-Brain-Pain' phenomenon.

After many years of treating patients with pain-related issues, I am certain of the value and importance of providing temporary relief of pain through injections, manipulations, physical therapy, and short-term use of medication (preferably non-addictive ones). However, I also believe that physicians have a duty to educate and encourage people to become more self-aware, so that they feel comfortable and safe enough to search within themselves, in order to root out their hidden causes of stress, dysfunctional habits, and pain. In this way, pain will not become chronic or recurrent. By combining pain and stress education - what I call 'pain literacy' - with the appropriate and effective treatment of pain symptoms, we can make a dramatic impact on quality of life. If practiced on a wider scale, this combined approach would have a huge impact on reducing the worldwide opioid crisis and disrupt the pattern of escalating health care costs.

In this way, the physician takes on the role of healer, teacher and coach. We can provide the education and encouragement needed for patients to motivate themselves to make meaningful changes that will reduce the negative effects of a life lived out of balance.

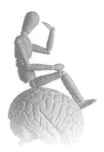

Chapter 2

The Brain on Pain

"Stress can wreak havoc on our metabolism, raise our blood
pressure, burst our white blood cells, make us flatulent,
ruin our sex life, and if that's not enough,
possibly damage our brain."

- Robert Sapolsky, *Why Zebras Don't Get Ulcers*

Pain as a Manifestation of Stress and the Threat Response

One of the central ideas of this book is that pain is a physical manifestation of stress. Negative emotions - such as anxiety, fear, anger, and rage - cause stress and trigger your brain's primitive threat response, sounding an alarm in the form of pain. This alarm is like the flashing 'check engine' light in your car. Your 'pain alarm' sends a ripple effect of electrochemical changes from the brain to your organs and tissues, as well as influencing your mood and behavior.

31

Below is a graphic illustration of how stress can affect our ability to function and stay healthy. Moreover, it demonstrates how we all have a tipping point, beyond which 'dis-stress,' dysfunction, and pain occur.

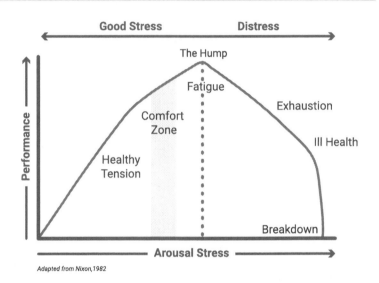

THE HUMAN FUNCTION CURVE

Adapted from Nixon,1982

There are three key takeaways in this chapter - learning how to recognize the early effects of fear and stress, taking conscious control of your threat response, and learning radical self-care. These insights are what you'll need to empower you to outsmart your pain and avoid becoming victim of your circumstances and old mental habits.

In this chapter, you'll learn that your pain patterns start and end in the brain, regardless of where your pain is experienced in the body. Therefore, you have many opportunities to change them.

Stress is unhelpful when:

- We can't cope, and we feel exhausted.
- We can't concentrate.
- We can't find the 'off' switch.
- We withdraw socially.
- We experience aches and pains and tension in our muscles.
- We have difficulty eating and sleeping.
- We become ungrounded.
- We feel anxious and distressed when facing difficult situations.

As you read this chapter, you'll discover how stress and other negative emotional states are connected and how they cause pain. Hopefully, you'll gain valuable information about recognizing the early warning signs of stress, before it leaves its indelible fingerprint on you in the form of pain and other health issues. We'll explore the effects of stress from your brain and body all the way down to the very tips of your DNA. Lastly, we'll discuss how you can effectively learn to cope with stress and identify steps that you can take to proactively prevent pain.

Your Emotional Nervous System

Your 'emotional nervous system' manages stress through the interaction of the brain via the 'limbic' system and autonomic nervous systems. This interaction establishes the framework of the mind-body connection, tying together the 'thinking' mind with the 'feeling' body. British psychologist Dr. Paul Gilbert, the founder of compassion focused therapy (CFT), developed a system to understand how people regulate emotions and manage stress. The focus of CFT is to teach gentle mind training techniques that help people work with experiences of feeling safe and to teach self soothing and self-compassion. According to Dr. Gilbert, your brain essentially switches between three different sub-systems, which include:

- The Drive Sub-System, which motivates you toward your desires and goals, but can lead to perfectionism, burnout, and depression. It is controlled by dopamine.
- The Soothing Sub-System, which manages 'di-stress,' by promoting self-healing, bonding, and relaxation. It is controlled by oxytocin and opiates.
- The Threat Sub-System, which is responsible for threat detection, protection, procreation, survival, and the 'better safe than sorry' mindset. It is controlled by adrenaline and cortisol.

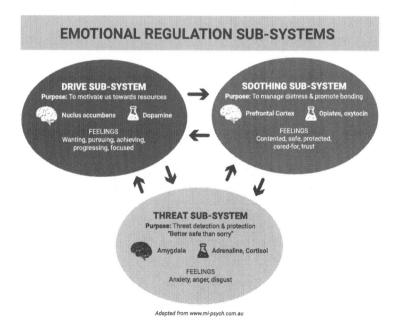

Adapted from www.mi-psych.com.au

If you're like most people, in daily life, you probably operate within a range between your threat and drive systems. We may not be the potential prey of wild animals anymore, but we are exposed to sensational news events, experience heavy traffic, have to manage work deadlines, balance family life, keep an eye on our finances, and much more. These daily stressors strain our threat and drive systems. This means that your soothing system could be under-functioning or even non-functional. Some people don't have time, but many people simply don't know how to self-soothe. Many people have never been taught or seen radical self-care in action, so they don't know what to do. We'll explore ideas about self-care and the soothing system later in the book.

'Eu-stress' or homeostasis is established when all three systems are in balance. In this ideal state, we can move from one system to another as needed. On the other hand, 'dis-tress' is caused by an imbalance between these three subsystems, and is usually the result of an under-functioning soothing system and over-functioning threat or drive systems.

When you predominantly balance between your threat and drive systems, you are swinging between the pendulum of extremes in your life, between aversion/pain and craving/pleasure. When it's not held in check by the other two systems, overemphasis of your drive system can lead to perfectionism, burnout, and addiction.

Threat-based emotions include fear, anger, and disgust. Our threat system identifies threats immediately, creating feelings of anxiety and fear in response to potentially threatening stimuli. These triggers create changes in your body chemistry and brain circuitry that motivate you to protect yourself, so you can feel safe.

The key point is that we are biased towards processing threat-based information. Our brains assign the highest threat value to pain, thereby triggering either the fight-or-flight response or submission. Furthermore, research shows that negative stimuli are more powerful signals to your brain than positive ones, taking hostage of your attention and thoughts. Additionally, due to your brain's ability to imagine, worry, and ruminate, it's possible for your threat system to be perpetually active over time, even in the absence of a genuine threat. This process is managed by the part of the brain called the limbic system.

The limbic system is often referred to as the 'paleo-mammalian brain.' The physical location of the limbic system is in the middle of the brain, between the two cerebral hemispheres and the brainstem. It is important because it allows us to make sense of our world. The limbic system evolved to manage the behavioral and emotional responses required for survival, including eating, reproduction, child-rearing, and the fight-or-flight response. All information that you experience from your five senses passes first through the amygdala, which sorts information from the limbic system into two categories: threat or non-threat. This input then stimulates the hypothalamus to trigger a fight-or-flight response.

Your limbic system has three components:

1. Hypothalamus
2. Hippocampus
3. Amygdala

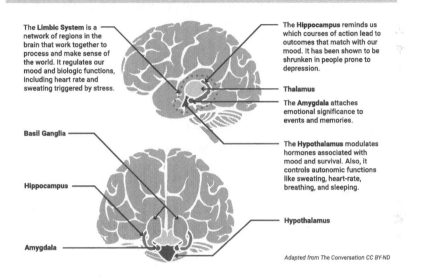

THE LIMBIC SYSTEM

The **Limbic System** is a network of regions in the brain that work together to process and make sense of the world. It regulates our mood and biologic functions, including heart rate and sweating triggered by stress.

The **Hippocampus** reminds us which courses of action lead to outcomes that match with our mood. It has been shown to be shrunken in people prone to depression.

Thalamus

The **Amygdala** attaches emotional significance to events and memories.

Basil Ganglia

The **Hypothalamus** modulates hormones associated with mood and survival. Also, it controls autonomic functions like sweating, heart-rate, breathing, and sleeping.

Hippocampus

Hypothalamus

Amygdala

Adapted from The Conversation CC BY-ND

We'll now explore how stress and the threat response affect these areas of the brain. First, pain is processed by an interactive network of five to ten areas of the brain. These areas constantly send information back and forth. These circuits are also responsible for the perception and modulation of pain. Chronic pain is now believed to be the result of faulty programming in these systems. Triggering events - such as stress, trauma, and injury - catalyze these processes. Sometimes, trigger events can occur long before we actually have pain, even by years or decades, making it difficult to connect the pain to its cause. We call these triggers 'antecedents' or 'pre-existing conditions.' These trigger events can predate the onset of pain, working evasively under the surface of our awareness, making it difficult to identify the source of our pain. Negative memories, fear, and anticipation of future symptoms (major flare-ups) stored in the amygdala can all be triggers with the profound ability to amplify pain via these circuits. They create neural pathways that operate beneath our conscious control.

Unlocking Fear and Its Hold on Our Muscles

Stress from a variety of sources, as well as fear, are perceived by your brain as threats, igniting identical threat responses in your body. Because your fight-or-flight response is designed to prime your muscles for action, when the stress/threat/fear response is over, your parasympathetic nervous system (PNS) should activate and instruct your muscles to relax. When you are stuck in stress/threat/fear mode, then your sympathetic nervous system (SNS) switch is stuck 'on.' Your PNS cannot then complete the task of facilitating your body to rest, digest, and repair itself, if it's cycling between real versus imagined threats. This is what leads to holding fear-based muscle tension patterns in your muscles. I'm sure that you (or someone you know well) has experienced neck and shoulder pain that makes you feel as though you're carrying the weight of the world on your shoulders.

Interestingly, even when your SNS switch is stuck in active mode, when you exercise vigorously, you can discharge excess cortisol and adrenaline, allowing for some level of muscle relaxation. However, this strategy doesn't allow tissues and cells to rest and repair. When people exclusively manage excess stress in this way by over-exercising, they may pay the price of frequent overuse injuries and overexertion. However, many of my patients are at the opposite end of that spectrum, saying that they are in too much pain to exercise, which presents a different conundrum: inertia!

So how does all of this work? Our fear/stress/threat response creates one of two muscle patterns. Either our muscles are primed and ready for action, or they seize up, creating a frozen state. Either state requires the PNS to release the tension once the threat is over.

Muscles are made up of many small fibers that combine into motor units, which are controlled by small motor nerves that are branches of a spinal nerve. When electrical impulses travel from the nerve to the muscle, the muscle unit has to respond with either contraction or relaxation. This is truly an all-or-nothing response; there is no middle ground. Without a signal to relax, your muscles stay contracted and the fear/stress/threat response essentially becomes 'trapped' in your muscles. During the fear/stress/threat response, your body is flooded with a burst of energy. If you stay stuck in tensed postures, without acting out or relaxing the 'energy,' it gets stuck inside your muscles. In a sense, your muscles are the end organ of the fear/stress/threat response circuit and everything gets bottlenecked there.

When muscle tension is finally released, so is the stuck 'energy.' This triggers the body to return to the same fear/stress/threat or hyperarousal mode that it was in when the threat response was originally initiated. This can happen even years after the original threat exposure and the person may not even realize the connection between the pain and the original trauma. This is one possible explanation for post-traumatic stress disorder (PTSD) which is commonly associated with chronic pain.

Trauma is real! It gets under our skin and then reshapes our reality. It is believed that the current prevalence of PTSD in chronic pain patients is 35 percent, as compared to 3.5 percent in the general population.

We experience fear and anxiety from situations that once caused us pain. The hurt and fear from these experiences code certain neural pathways which then generate specific responses in our brain and autonomic nervous system. This way when we are exposed to similar situations in the future, we are reminded of the same danger and the fear response is re-activated, which triggers dysregulation of our nervous system, pain, and muscle tension. neuroscience researcher and author of The Polyvagal Theory, Dr. Stephen Porges and, has done much research on trauma and the 'quest for safety' and their effects on the nervous system.

"Fear does not stop death, it stops life."

- Vi Keeland

Stress and the Threat Response

Remember that stress is the result of the ways in which your brain and body respond to both real and perceived threats. It is estimated that 90 percent of all doctor visits are for stress-related health complaints. Imagine how things could change when the focus of healthcare becomes effective stress management, rather than just symptom and pain management.

Like pain, stress can be acute (short-term) or chronic (long-term). The non-stop elevation of stress hormones that occurs in chronic pain starts as a chain reaction of electrochemical events that results in a 'fight, flight, or freeze' response. This throws the body out of the desired state of homeostasis, disrupting the balance of the sympathetic nervous system (SNS) and the para-sympathetic nervous system (PNS). When this happens, there is suppression of your normal brain's ability to consciously over-ride the threat response. This 'unleashes the beast,' wreaking havoc on your health and causing inflammation, pain, and suffering.

THREATS

The brain does not know the difference.
It is only concerned with one thing:

IS THIS A THREAT?

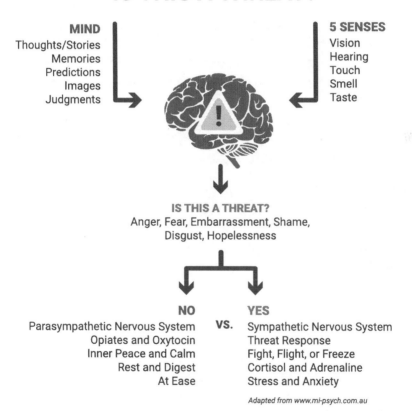

MIND	5 SENSES
Thoughts/Stories	Vision
Memories	Hearing
Predictions	Touch
Images	Smell
Judgments	Taste

IS THIS A THREAT?
Anger, Fear, Embarrassment, Shame,
Disgust, Hopelessness

NO	**vs.**	**YES**
Parasympathetic Nervous System		Sympathetic Nervous System
Opiates and Oxytocin		Threat Response
Inner Peace and Calm		Fight, Flight, or Freeze
Rest and Digest		Cortisol and Adrenaline
At Ease		Stress and Anxiety

Adapted from www.mi-psych.com.au

This threat response is hardwired into the brain and has always been part of our evolutionary survival mechanism. We are all designed to handle bite-sized pieces of stress and transient

41

negative emotions. However, we are not typically equipped to handle the chronic long-term effects of stress and negative emotional states. While it's true that some people are better equipped to handle stress, each of us has a different threshold or tolerance. Studies even show that men and women handle stress differently. Women's stress hormone receptors are less adaptive than men's, making women more susceptible to the harmful effects of stress.

Furthermore, similar findings have been reported in terms of how women handle pain. Dr. Jeffrey Mogil of McGill University has shown that women are more sensitive to pain than men. Women typically rate their pain higher than men on the subjective zero to ten scale. It is not known whether this is a purely genetic factor or in part a behavioral one. He further states that empathy can make pain worse and suggests that this may explain some of the differences between men and women.

Empathy is our ability to understand and share the feelings of another. it is generally considered a trait of evolved people. In a sense, we are wired for empathy through the effects of 'mirror neurons' in our brain. You could consider the idea that there is a scale of empathy between healthy empathy and extreme empathy with the later leading to enabling and enmeshment, rather than empowerment.

Paul Bloom in his book, *Against Empathy*, explains that empathy is different from compassion and can lead to more pain. Researchers Tania Singer and Olga Klimecki argue that, "in contrast to empathy, compassion does not mean sharing the suffering of the other; rather it is characterized by feelings of warmth, concern and care for the other, as well as strong motivation to improve the other's wellbeing. Compassion is feeling for and not feeling with the other." In my view, empathy focuses on the problem and compassion is concern expressed through the lens of how to help the other improve their condition. In other words, compassion is solution-focused rather than problem-focused social engagement.

I am reminded of a male patient in his mid thirties, who came to see me with mysterious left hip pain and what he described as 'burning mouth syndrome.' When we talked about his life, he described how he takes on all of the suffering of those he loves. His wife confirmed this at his initial visit. Further, she shared that she had suffered with a long history of migraine headaches before she met him. Once he took on her suffering, her headaches went away. He is so empathic that his behavior borders on a martyr complex. Interestingly, he doesn't come from a place of guilt, but more from a place of love. He doesn't know how to be compassionate without taking on everyone else's negative 'stuff.' This is the dark side of empathy. During his physical exam, I wasn't surprised to find tattoos of Jesus Christ, accompanied by other black-and-white body art with vivid images of mortal pain and suffering.

Clearly, this is an extreme case, but many people are empathic to an extreme, and they are unaware of how this negatively impacts their health and wellbeing. Letting go of what is not ours to bear is important to being emotionally and physically healthy. It allows us to better manage our stress levels and keeps our nervous system from getting overloaded.

The human condition is clearly a delicate one. For better or worse, we are influenced by those around us. We learn how to handle stress and relate to pain from those closest to us. Studies reveal that various early life experiences impact our ability to handle stress later in life. When you're exposed to the trauma of neglect and abusive situations, you become sensitized to stress. You may block out the stress as a way of avoiding 'overwhelm' and burnout, but this may make you vulnerable to developing a hair trigger for even the slightest fearful things down the road. These triggers are unique to all of us. We learn how to handle stress and relate to pain from those closest to us.

This means that some of your early experiences can actually become triggers for the threat response and contribute to pain later in life. As we age, these adverse childhood experiences (ACE) are significant risk factors for chronic pain and many chronic illnesses. As you'll discover in Chapter 3, neuroplasticity has a significant impact on how your brain is wired.

Due to the effects of neural grooves, which create recurring patterns of thought and behavior, you continue to think and do the same old things, until you consciously choose to change them. Old patterns even from childhood tend to persist without our conscious awareness. Making conscious changes takes awareness and effort because you must get out of the rut or groove created by neural plasticity in the brain. The good news is that there are things you can do to influence your stress level and reduce pain, including:

- Strengthen your support network. Supportive (compassionate) family and friends are a great buffer against stress.
- Learn how to soothe yourself. This could include relaxing activities such as a movie night, massage, being in nature, or day at the spa.
- Be prepared ahead of time, so that you leave less to chance, which may mitigate your reactions to stressful situations in the heat of the moment.
- Have a positive attitude and maintain your sense of humor.

- Have confidence and faith that only good things will happen. This gives you a 'sense of control' over the situation so that you don't feel like a victim.

The On/Off Switch

Your stress or threat response is designed to be turned 'on' when absolutely needed, and then turned 'off' when the threat is over. Most of us are unaware of this on/off switch. Without that knowledge, we are unable to flip the switch to shut the threat response off. You can probably see how this primitive threat/warning system helped when our ancestors survived threats ranging from wild animal attacks to natural disasters. In our modern world, this threat response is harder to recognize and manage, because our stressors are more insidious. After all, we don't have saber-toothed tigers chasing us anymore.

Today, our stressors tend to sneak up on us, causing us to feel frazzled, hijacking small chunks of our health and state of mind, until we become sick or suffer from pain. Additionally, the negative effects of stress impact our immune system, leaving us more vulnerable to illness and more susceptible to harm. Once you fully understand this as the essential function of our psychoneuroimmunology, and decide to take self-responsibility for making changes to mitigate these effects, the healthier you'll be.

The first step in controlling stress is to recognize its symptoms. This may be harder than you think, because most of us are so accustomed to living in constant stress. How many people do you know that seem to brag about 'how busy they are' or constantly bemoan 'how stressed they are'? Most of us have become numb to the early warning signs. We often fail to take notice, until we're in so much 'dis-tress' and pain that we reach our breaking point and finally seek medical help.

Returning to the ideas from Chapter 1, stress, and one of its many physical manifestations, pain, are modulated by your brain and nervous system through the release of electrical and chemical signals. Some of the the key players have already been identified as the limbic system (brain), spinal cord and autonomic nervous system. Now, we will address the adrenal glands, which produce the hormone cortisol.

The Electrochemical Stress Response

There are three main components in the body that control the electrochemical stress or threat response: the hypothalamus and pituitary gland (both in your brain), and your adrenal glands (small glands sitting on top of the kidneys). The sequence of events is as follows. Your brain perceives danger, sending immediate electrochemical signals down your spinal cord to your adrenal glands, instructing them to release adrenaline and cortisol. Adrenaline then triggers an increase of sugar (glucose) in your blood, giving you energy to mount a fight-or-flight response. This is when your muscles tighten, your senses sharpen, and your heart starts to beat faster, with blood flow increasing - by a factor of three to four times - to prepare your legs, lungs, and brain for fighting the threat or running to safety.

While this is happening other major body systems shut down - including your GI tract - as they are considered non-essential during stressful events. As cortisol rises, it keeps your blood sugar and blood pressure elevated to support your fight-or-flight response, which wreaks havoc on other systems, leading to a pro-inflammatory state within your body. This is exacerbated when the stress/threat mechanism fails to shut off properly and cortisol levels climb out of control. This is why many healthcare professionals consider cortisol to be 'public enemy number one!'

THE ACTH AXIS

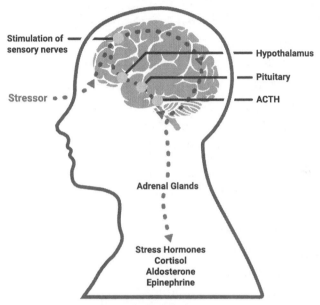

Stimulation of sensory nerves

Hypothalamus

Pituitary

Stressor

ACTH

Adrenal Glands

Stress Hormones
Cortisol
Aldosterone
Epinephrine

THE STRESS RESPONSE

Increased neural excitability
Increased cardiovascular activity
   Heart rate, stroke volume, cardiac
   output, blood pressure
Increased metabolic activity
   Gluconeogenesis:
      Turning glycogen into
      sugar for energy
   Protein mobilization:
      Decreased antibody producer
      Muscle wasting
   Fat mobilization:
      For breakdown into sugar
Increased sodium retention (salt)
Increase in neurological sweating
Change in salivation
Change in GI system tonus and motility

Adapted from *Physiology of Stress*, Jones and Bartlett Publishers

Cortisol production in the body has a natural circadian rhythm, with the lowest levels at night and the highest levels in the morning. Another element involved in our circadian rhythm is the autonomic nervous system. When we sleep, it's crucial that our cortisol levels are reduced, so can we activate our parasympathetic nervous system, resulting in muscle relaxation, deeper breathing, resetting of our hormones, and so on. This physiologic reset is designed to restore homeostasis each night. Otherwise, we remain stuck in the stress/threat response. Anything that interferes with our sleep and this natural rest-and-reset period can short circuit the system, prolonging the threat response.

People can also get stuck in a parasympathetic state or a sympathetic state. People stuck in PNS states are typically depressed, lethargic, dissociated, and they present with low blood pressure. People stuck in SNS states are just the opposite. They are anxious, hyper-vigilant, tired, and sleepless, suffer from Attention Deficit Disorder (ADD) or Obsessive Compulsive Disorder (OCD), and are typically agitated and angry.

Three factors that are relevant today in managing stress and optimizing health. First is the overall strength of our nervous system. Second is the equilibrium between excitation (SNS) and inhibition (PNS). Third is our conscious capacity and willingness to switch between these two states. Taking all of this into consideration can dramatically improve the way we manage stress, reduce pain and suffering, and alter the impact of chronic disease in our lives.

Stress Effects on the Brain

Research shows the release of adrenaline and cortisol in the bloodstream are critical for mounting our escape from threatening situations. If these hormones stay elevated for more than a couple of weeks, they start to impair our immune system. This chain of events can also result in premature brain aging, due to the loss of brain cells in the two important parts of the brain: the hippocampus (where memories are stored) and the prefrontal cortex (which affects decision making and behavior control). This phenomenon will also lead to the impairment of cognitive function, problem solving, creativity, and memory.

Our hippocampus is also responsible for shutting off the stress response when the immediate threat is over. This is an area we need to function well, because it's part of the 'off' switch. If the threat response doesn't shut off, and the body remains primed for fight-or-flight without engaging in any action, then these stress hormones start running amok, which can cause inflammation and pain and short-circuit our organ systems. This will also impact our ability to take in new information and make good choices.

Stress and heightened threat response patterns also cause 'free radicals' to form in the brain. Free radicals are free-floating oxygen molecules that break down the integrity of the blood-brain barrier, causing what I refer to as 'leaky brain.' This condition is similar to the concept of 'leaky gut,' which causes undigested food particles, toxic waste products, and bacteria to 'leak' through a damaged small intestine lining, flooding the bloodstream, and harming the tissues. This can explain many chronic degenerative nervous system conditions.

In addition, many neurotransmitters and chemicals in the brain are affected by stress. Brain-derived neurotrophic factor (BDNF), which is a protective substance in the brain, decreases when your cortisol levels rise. Stress and threat have similar effects on two other neurotransmitters: serotonin (the happy molecule) and dopamine (the motivation and addiction molecule).

Stress also increases the size and activity of another limbic system structure - the amygdala - which makes you more fearful, causing you to be more susceptible to the stress/threat effect. Additionally, within the brain is a 'mini-immune system' operated by cells called microglia. Stress activates your microglial cells, producing inflammation in the brain.

In my patients, I see that inflammation caused by elevated cortisol levels can result in pain virtually anywhere in the body. Functional Medicine has a special role in helping us assess pain and disease caused by inflammation. This is particularly true for stress-related gut issues that generate inflammation, which can affect any part of your body. Remember that stress rewires your brain, leaving you more susceptible to mood disorders, such as depression and anxiety.

Stress and Anxiety

There are three important distinctions between stress and anxiety. First, anxiety persists long after the stressor is gone. Second, anxiety is anticipatory and is usually based on an imagined threat. Third, anxiety is often accompanied by a persistent feeling of worry, apprehension, or dread. Anxiety creates a short circuit in your ability to balance your 'emotional nervous system.'

The best way to deal with anxiety is recognize its causes and develop the tools and mechanisms to help you cope effectively, rather than taking potentially addictive medications that will further impair your ability to think clearly. Slowly untangling the various factors driving your threat system will help tremendously. Can you think of factors that make you fearful? It's a good idea to write them down, start to process them, and be able to get them out of your head. Tens of millions of people struggling with anxiety would benefit from learning these ideas. This is one of many things that inspired me to write this book!

Stress Triggers

Keep in mind if you get 'stressed out' easily, as many in our hectic world do, you may be in a heightened state of stress much of the time, without being aware of it. What triggers stress, and ultimately what causes pain, depends on your perception of it. Your past exposures are also very important triggers. We all have various external causes of stress, such as the loss of a job or an important relationship, financial struggles, and illness and death of loved ones. Some internal stressors include an intolerance of uncertainty, fear of the unknown, constant worrying, rigid all-or-nothing thinking, unrealistic expectations, perfectionism, and negative self-talk.

Other Manifestations of Stress

Remember that 90 percent of all primary care visits are due to stress-related problems. Nearly one-half of all American adults suffer from the adverse effects of stress. Chronic stress speeds up the aging process, affects our DNA and disrupts many of your organ systems. It also impacts your digestive, cardiovascular, and reproductive systems, as well as your mental and emotional health.

Other health problems linked to stress and the threat response are:

- Pain of any kind
- Weight gain and obesity
- Headaches
- Sleep problems, including insomnia
- Digestive issues, such as irritable bowel syndrome and reflux

- Skin conditions, including eczema and psoriasis
- Autoimmune conditions
- Cardiovascular disease
- Hypertension
- Reproductive issues and sexual dysfunction (including loss of sex drive)
- Memory issues
- Attention Deficit Disorder (ADD)
- Constant worrying and obsessive thinking
- Irritability
- Self-criticism
- Anger
- Memory issues
- Frequent colds

Some steps to manage stress more effectively include:

- Become clear about the source of your stress, whether it is relationships, work, finances, perfectionism, fear, and so on.
- Open up and express your thoughts and feelings instead of keeping them bottled inside. This can be achieved through journaling or working with a coach or therapist.
- Simplify your life by clarifying your priorities. Start making yourself and your health your the top priority.
- Recognize the effects that food, alcohol, caffeine, and drugs have on your state of balance and wellbeing.
- Set boundaries and learn how to say 'no.'
- Find recreational activities that you enjoy.
- Find a healthy balance of activity, relaxation, and rest.

- Keep a diary or journal of stressful situations and events in your life. Record your emotions and physical symptoms. This can help you connect the dots.
- Learn mind-body practices - such as breathing exercises, meditation, yoga, and biofeedback - that help you connect with how you feel and function.

Taking Care of Yourself

Learning to manage stress is critical for your health. There are two basic stress-coping strategies. One approach targets your challenging thoughts and emotions, while the other revolves around actual problem-solving the lifestyle issues that contribute to stress.

You can achieve homeostasis in many ways. A balanced lifestyle includes: good nutrition, proper exercise, learning self-soothing techniques, regular relaxation, having fun, diaphragmatic (deep) breathing, journaling, prayer, and meditation. Another key element of healing your brain from stress is to kill the 'ANTS' (automatic negative thoughts), which was originally described by Dr. Daniel Amen in his book *Change Your Brain, Change Your Life*. ANTS are the negative thoughts, that as Dr. Amen says, "invade your mind like ants at a picnic," triggering the threat response and increasing cortisol production. Stress can also be a sign that we're compromising what's good for us individually to satisfy the needs of others, sacrificing our own needs in the process.

It's important to recognize that self-care is different than selfishness. When we're in relationships with others, it's challenging to balance our own needs with their needs. Learning to recognize your needs, and having them sufficiently met, are essential to a happy and fulfilling life.

Like many of us, you have probably witnessed or experienced dysfunctional relationship models throughout your life. Some people may even lack a single point of reference for what a healthy, balanced relationship looks like. Relationships based on an unrealistic imbalance of others' needs being met, while yours are ignored, become codependent, rather than interdependent. As you can imagine, this common dysfunctional relationship pattern causes considerable stress, pain, and suffering.

If you can identify part of your story in these passages, I urge you to take stock and reevaluate your needs and assess how you will experience joy; find your special place of comfort and peace in your world, where you are supported and 'stress-free.'

In the next chapter, you will learn how the brain can trick us, keeping us stuck, exacerbating our stress, and preventing us from achieving this ideal state of mind and way of life.

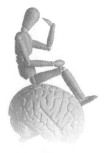

Chapter 3

'We Are Wired for Pain'
- The Role of Neuroplasticity

"The feel is real, but the why is a lie."

- Guy Finley

Neuroplasticity

The concept of neuroplasticity refers to your brain's capacity to physically reorganize itself throughout your entire lifetime. Think of how plastic can change under different temperature conditions. Your brain is much the same. In a healthy brain, all regions exist in a state of integration or equilibrium, which is referred to as the brain's 'resting state network.' This means that all parts of your brain work equally, contributing to one functioning whole.

New neuronal connections in the brain constantly form in response to external and internal stimuli. Your health status, behavior, thoughts, emotions, relationships, and physical surroundings all affect your brain's capacity to evolve and meet new challenges. Neuroplasticity is remarkable because it forms the physiological basis for the possibility of growth, learning, and change. However, it also forms habitual grooves in our thinking and behavior when our thoughts and emotions are negative. According to Dr. Kim and Dr. Hil of Authenticity Associates, "most people live on autopilot most of the time. This is because neural pathways operate under the law of least effort and therefore follow the path of least resistance."

Important Facts about Neuroplasticity:

People of any age can learn and develop new habits and skills. When we get into a rut and stop exercising, become too sedentary, or develop poor eating habits, the principle of neuroplasticity gives us the power to make changes, if that's our goal.

We can train our brain and build it up like a muscle. This process transcends simple behavioral changes, adaptations, and learning. It means that your brain can actually rewire itself. In doing so, the gray matter in your brain physically changes.

In exercising your brain power on a regular basis, you can build reserve brain function to draw upon at moments of need. However, be aware that stress affects neuroplasticity by destroying neurons and neuronal connections. It is nearly impossible to live without stress, but how we manage our stress is critical to the growth or depletion of our brain power.

Neuroplasticity and Pain

Because chronic pain is 'learned' pain, it can change and damage your brain, affecting everything from mental processing speed to mood and memory. Pain disturbs the balance of your brain as a whole, making it harder for you to make good decisions. Research shows that the long-term effects of chronic low back pain include actual shrinkage of the hippocampus, the part of the brain responsible for your mental performance, learning, and memory. Memory, imagination, and perception are three different software processes that run on the same platform in the brain, and it is not yet clear how pain affects the latter two. As you will see in the diagram below from Dr. Michael Moskowitz and Dr. Marla DePolo Golden's book, *Neuroplastic Transformation: Your Brain on Pain,* chronic pain starts to take over important 'real estate' in the brain.

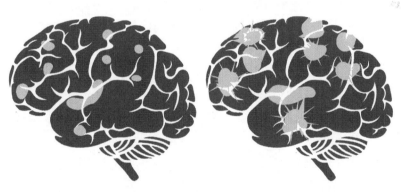

PAIN MAPS

Acute Pain Perception   **Persistent Pain Perception**

In persistent pain, the brain pain map expands up to 5 times.
THE BRAIN LEARNS PAIN

Adapted from neuroplastix.com

Chronic pain has been shown to age your brain by making it harder to learn new information and engage in appropriate emotional regulation. Another area affected by chronic pain is the amygdala, which is an area of the brain important for fear regulation and emotion-related memory tasks. The effects of pain on the amygdala lead to increased anxiety. As such, chronic pain not only causes shrinkage of neurons in these key areas of the brain, but also results in compensation by other parts of the brain. This compensation pattern puts healthy neurons in other parts of the brain under strain, causing an already malfunctioning brain additional emotional frustration, potentially influencing one's responsiveness to conventional pain treatments.

As such, it's important to be open to a variety of pain therapies that may help to prevent your chronic pain from having such a negative impact on your brain. This means that treating pain is not as simple as prescribing analgesic pain-relieving drugs or anti-inflammatories. It opens up room to consider other helpful treatment modalities including:

- Interventional pain treatments
- Physical therapy
- Cognitive Behavioral Therapies (CBT) and Compassion Focused Therapy (CFT)
- Acupuncture
- Massage
- Reflexology
- Hypnotherapy
- Yoga
- Mindfulness
- Energy work

CBT is a form of counseling aimed at reducing the perception of pain as well as reducing maladaptive thoughts and attitudes that contribute to pain. The goal of CBT is to reduce feelings of helplessness, build a sense of control over pain, and learn better coping strategies. On the other hand, CFT helps us learn to balance our emotional subsystems and become more compassionate with ourselves and others. These modalities will be discussed further in Chapter 7 - The Pain Treatment Tool Box.

Earlier in this chapter, I discussed how neuroplasticity can work for us or against us. I want to emphasize that, while your brain undergoes these physical and functional changes in response to pain, the changes are reversible. Once the pain is treated effectively, without the influence of strong opioid pain medications, the mind and body can be restored to equilibrium.

Neuroplasticity and the Physical Body

Your brain and nervous system are adaptable and constantly changing based on input from various sources. Neuroplasticity also has vast effects on the body, because the brain can unlearn and relearn proper and improper movement patterns. Unfortunately, when we adopt distorted body postures and altered movement patterns due to pain, our brains eventually establish a 'new normal.' These compensatory changes result in totally inefficient movement patterns that lead to muscle fatigue, muscle spasms, and pain due to overuse. Then, these patterns form well-worn grooves that, over time, have a significant impact on your muscles, tendons, ligaments, posture, and gait.

These protective responses distort posture and stimulate (upregulate) the sympathetic nervous system, causing manifestations of stress and anxiety. The effects of these compensatory changes are usually not obvious, and unfortunately, they don't show up on standard X-rays, MRIs, or CAT scans. I frequently see patients in my office who appear to have seemingly normal gait patterns, but when I look at their tendon attachments, I see numerous bone spurs. I explain to them that the tendons are similar to puppet strings. Where the strings attach, stress points occur in the form of bone spurs and tendon calcifications.

This is especially true if the 'puppet' is biased to one side, with the string on one side under more tension than the other. These kinds of compensation patterns are very common and can cause a considerable amount of pain. I see this most often in the shoulder and hip as they are both 'ball and socket' joints. When there's an imbalanced pull of the tendons around the ball then it doesn't seat properly in the joint, leading to premature breakdown of the tendons, as well as cartilage and bones. Sometimes gait deviations can be so subtle that a physician and physical therapist may not be able to identify them with the naked eye. Computerized gait analysis can be helpful in these circumstances. Seeking help from a physical therapist with specialized training in muscle re-education techniques such as Dynamic Neuromuscular Stabilization (DNS) or Postural Restoration (PRI) will be helpful in breaking these dysfunctional patterns. This will be discussed in Chapter 7 - The Pain Treatment Tool Box.

Neuroplasticity and the Brain

The human brain is made up of approximately 100 billion neurons, which combine to form 100 trillion neuronal connections. These are designed to ensure your survival and maintain homeostasis. Neuroplasticity forms the basis of change and transformation. Rewiring your brain is a dynamic process that happens within the relationship of your mind, brain, and body.

The prefrontal cortex is prime real estate in the brain, especially when it comes to making conscious changes that reduce pain and improve feelings of happiness and well-being. Strengthening activity in the prefrontal cortex has many positive effects, including releasing the feel-good chemical serotonin, making it easier to replicate feelings of happiness and overriding negative default programs.

As we'll discuss in the next chapter, you should avoid 'practicing your pain' or making it a habit. This is because focusing on pain can embed it in your brain. This process, called 'pain imprinting,' leads to electrical and chemical changes in the body that reinforce the pain pathways in the brain. As your pain persists, the neural grooves deepen, becoming a powerful force to reckon with. Unfortunately, your brain likes that which is known, often defaulting to making the same poor choices, unless you consciously override them. According to Drs. Kim and Hil, "Once you know how to develop and strengthen neural pathways, you can change just about anything you want."

Here are some of the ways you can reprogram your brain to reduce pain:

- Know your pain triggers (see Chapter 5).
- Pay attention and cultivate self-awareness. This helps activate your prefrontal cortex, which is a good thing!
- Make small changes to reduce pain and celebrate your successes. Changing behavior releases serotonin and helps grow your willpower muscles.
- Surround yourself with positive people who support your goals.
- Storyboard your journey to pain relief.
- Learn how to use the 'recovery loop' to change the 'habit loop' (presented in Chapter 4). The brain learns to enjoy recovery and those things that give you meaning and pleasure.

- Consciously redirect your mind to get rid of old negative thoughts and practice new ways of thinking.
- Practice positivity. Practice doing something every day that you enjoy.
- Declare your goals by stating them out loud every morning.
- Visualize being pain-free and living the life of your dreams.
- Meditate to calm the mind and reduce stress. When we are stressed, our brain automatically defers to the strongest neural pathway. This is part of our innate survival mechanism. This is the 'path of least resistance.'
- Manage your energy resources wisely. Learn to say 'no' when other people's agendas interfere with your own needs.
- Practice self-soothing and self-care (such techniques will be presented in the final chapters).
- Connect with nature. It grounds you, so you don't short circuit.

Neuroplasticity and Your Genes

According to the Visual Meditation Company, "You 'speak' to your genes with every thought you have." Epigenetics is the science of how your genes can be switched on or off by your choices and life experiences.

It is believed that 95 percent of our 22 thousand genes are influenced by, and can influence, lifestyle factors such as sleep, nutrition, exercise, and stress management. At least 4 thousand genes have been identified by genetics researchers as influencing our experience of pain. Soon, genetic testing will be more readily available to assess possible genetic vulnerability to certain types of pain. Another influence on your genetic expression is exposure to challenging or traumatic life experiences, including adverse childhood events, such as abuse, abandonment, neglect, and substance abuse. Studies show that people exposed to these early life traumas are more likely than their age-matched peers to develop chronic pain and chronic disease. If you have a high Adverse Childhood Event (ACE) score, then exploring this as a pain trigger may be helpful. If you are not sure if this applies to you, you can take the test online and explore this concept further at *www. acestudy.org.*

My sister, Dr. Shelley Binder, a professor at The University of Tennessee, has been studying the effects of trauma on subsequent generations of a family. In the case of our own family, our great grandmother, Leah Aks, was a third class passenger aboard the maiden and only voyage of the Titanic, which of course, sunk tragically after striking an iceberg on April 14, 1912. My family has always been fascinated by the amazing events that took place that night and the fact that our then 17 year-old grandmother and the infant in her arms were able to survive. This story has become our family story. Shelley has been particularly interested in exploring what happened to the Titanic's survivors. She even teaches a college course on the topic.

Shelley spent many years unraveling many stories and myths to develop a deeper understanding of the truth of these events. She has done an incredible amount of research, digging into all sorts of historical records of the actual traumas that occured that night in 1912. She has also investigated records of how the survivors were received in New York City and how they were treated afterward. What she has uncovered is that the survivors experienced considerable PTSD and survivor guilt.

There is now growing evidence that traumas such as these can live on in future generations, as a result of epigenetic effects.

63

I can't help but wonder if some of us are wired to be 'survivors' and others are not? Do these sorts of family experiences potentially impact genetic factors that determine our stress response patterns and predetermine our psychoneuroimmunology? Interestingly, Native American folklore teaches the "Seventh Generation Principle" which hypothesizes that every decision we make, and every event in our lives, can affect our descendants seven generations into the future. This idea has far reaching implications for us to all consider.

What happened to you or your family in the past (especially what was beyond your control) has shaped your brain, programmed your cells, and switched on or off certain genes. However, you always have the power to choose your perspective and behavior in the present and future.

As you learned in Chapter 2, your ability to self-regulate stress and manage your emotional state is directly dependent on your thoughts. Epigenetics shows that your perceptions and thoughts have more of an influence over your biology than the other way around. The link between epigenetics and lifestyle is further proof of the mind-body connection. This is good news, because it means you pivot your negative thoughts into positive ones, and outsmart your genes to optimize your health.

Vision Board Your Pain-Free Life

Consider creating a vision board of how you want to feel, what you want to do, and where you want to go. You can do this by drawing pictures or clipping images that fit how you feel and see yourself now on the left side of the paper; and then draw a line down the middle of the page. On the right side of the paper, create images of how you would like to feel and what you want your life to look like. Then, as pain physician and author Dr.

Peter Abaci describes, draw a bridge between the two sides (where you are now on the left and where you want to be on the right).

Once your vision is clear, then you can start identifying the right habits you'll need to cross over that bridge. If you get stuck, then you can take another piece of paper and write on the left-hand side all the habits that work against your vision of a better life. And on the right side, write down the specific habit(s) you want to adopt. Think of these as the health habits that will help you make the pivot to a pain free life.

Sometimes it's helpful to explore the stories of people who have transformed their lives through neuroplasticity. Connecting with others who have made positive changes in their lives is wonderful. However, I would caution you against chronic pain chat rooms and some online support groups in which people focus on their problems, rather than appropriate helpful solutions. We all know that misery loves company. However, I urge you not to waste your time feeling sorry for yourself or others. This can take you to the dark side of empathy and activate the negative default pathways that will keep you stuck in pain.

FEELING VISION BOARD

HOW DO YOU FEEL NOW?	HOW DO YOU WANT TO FEEL?
1.	1.
2.	2.
3.	3.
4.	4.
5.	5.

HABITS VISION BOARD

HABITS WORKING AGAINST YOU	HABITS WORKING FOR YOU
1.	1.
2.	2.
3.	3.
4.	4.
5.	5.

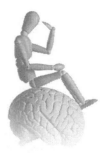

Chapter 4

Pain as a Habit

**"If you change the way you look at things,
the things you look at change."**

- Wayne Dyer

Your pain is created by a host of physical events, memories of past experiences, thoughts, fears, and emotions. Your pain is also a product of your unique physiology and biochemistry. However, pain can also become a habit. It's a learned behavior and not just a response to a physical injury. As such, you can outsmart it. To do so successfully, you need to address your pain habits and change them. It's that simple, yet so many who suffer struggle to do so.

Do you know someone whose life revolves around their pain? These folks practice their pain habits on a regular basis by focusing on them and broadcasting them to the world. They take potentially harmful medications, often with little or only modest benefit. They see countless doctors and specialists and complain when they don't find solutions. Instead of working toward a solution, they incessantly worry about their condition. They allow their pain to fill every thought, action, and conversation. Because of their pain, they limit their activities, alienate their loved ones, and focus on what they can't do. As a consequence, all of these behaviors continually remind their brain of pain. They constantly form negative thought loops about their pain, creating triggers in the form of specific activities or behaviors that keep the pain habit going.

In the field of pain medicine, we even see some people with chronic pain 'give up.' Unfortunately, they become resigned to a sense of hopelessness, also called 'learned helplessness.' Studies show that, once a person reaches this state of desperation, and loses all sense of hope, their response to any treatment is limited. This is partly due to the neuronal connections that are formed in the brain, which are the basis for how these people habitually think and what they habitually do. It is also the result of exhaustion of one's energy resources. Due to the prolonged exposure to chronic pain and stress, one drops into the 'red zone,' with no gas left in the tank to keep going. This state represents a complete depletion of chemical, hormonal, and immunological functions of the HPA axis.

As you learned in the last chapter, neuroplasticity can work for or against us. We see this in people who take opioid medication to alleviate pain. Their brains become sensitized or 'cued' to the medication, and their brains begin to crave the drug. This is partly how drug addiction starts. The first time we do something, such as take a pill for pain, our brain releases the chemical dopamine, which immediately sends reward messages to the brain. Eventually, due to neuroplastic changes in the brain, dopamine gets released when we anticipate the action (before it actually happens). This motivates us to take the action - the pill - in the future. With practice, this pattern gets grooved into the nervous system, becoming the path of least resistance. This is one reason why many people who take opioids are resistant to new solutions for pain relief.

Habit 'Hacks'

In his book, *The Craving Mind,* psychiatrist Dr. Judson Brewer describes how mindfulness-based stress reduction (MBSR) techniques can help us to deal with cravings for medication or anything else that is habit-forming or addictive. He likens the process of dealing with cravings or habits to surfing the waves of wanting or craving using a Buddhist practice with the acronym RAIN. The first step of this practice is *recognizing* that the craving or wanting is coming, like it or not, and then *relaxing* into it. The next step is to *acknowledge* or *accept* the wave as it is, rather than ignoring it, trying to change it or play the distraction game. He notes that to catch the wave of wanting, you employ curiosity to study it carefully, *investigating* it as it builds. This allows you to take *note* of what you are thinking, as well as what is happening in your body in the moment. In other words, how do you feel? Is there a sensation in your stomach, burning or pain anywhere, or possibly a headache? If so follow it with you attention, until it completely subsides. After having studied MBSR with Dr. Brewer and his colleagues, I would encourage you to explore it either through an online training program or in-person courses. Either way, learning the skills of mindfulness is a sure way to outsmart your pain. These helpful techniques, and many others, will be discussed in more detail in Chapter 7 - The Pain Treatment Tool Box and Chapter 8 - Health as a Habit.

Habits, such as drug dependency, also form 'mental loops.' In his book, *The Power of Habit*, Charles Duhigg discusses how we can use what he calls the three-part habit loop to change our health and make our lives more meaningful. As you will learn, a habit loop consist of a cue, an action, and a reward.

His research demonstrates that it actually takes 66 days to form a new habit. He asserts that identifying clear cues, and tying them to meaningful rewards, are more effective than simply changing our actions. These cues and rewards are so important because, whenever we see the cue, our brain releases dopamine and we begin craving the reward. This means that as soon as we see the cue, the craving makes a new habit form automatically.

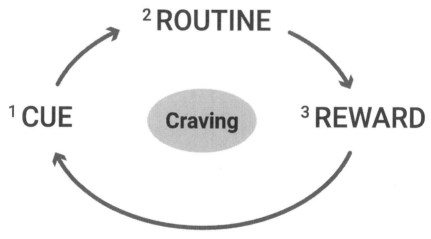

Adapted from Charles Duhigg

Habits can be pervasive and insidious, both from a mental and physical perspective. For example, patients who have prolonged hospital stays - where they're given laxatives nightly - develop a pattern where they believe they can't evacuate their bowels without the medication. It can take weeks to wean them back to a normal routine.

In the same way as pain medication - where the addiction rate is well known - almost anything can become an addictive habit. Overeating when one is not hungry is a classic example. Teaching people how to change their food choices, and embrace healthy nutrition almost always leads to significant weight loss, resulting in lower blood pressure, the prevention of diabetes, and the relief of pressure and pain in the back, knees, and joints. In theory, these positive benefits would seem to be reward enough. Not so. The siren call of food, with cravings far stronger than the rewards of health, is deafening for many people. Overcoming food addiction means boldly breaking the habit loop.

Now that we see how habits are formed and perpetuated, we can explore other reasons that pain can become a habit.

1. Poor Posture
2. Poor Body Awareness
3. Poor Breathing Patterns
4. Lack of Grounding
5. Poor Sleep Hygiene
6. Poor Nutrition
7. Perfectionism
8. Overthinking Pain

You will explore each of these topics throughout this chapter. Additional mental and emotional habits considered as risk factors for chronic pain also deserve a mention, including

- Staying stuck in the past and resistance to change.
- Holding onto negative thoughts and emotions.
- Early life trauma that has been blocked.
- Emotional numbing or dissociation

Let's explore the factors that can increase or decrease the risk of developing chronic pain:

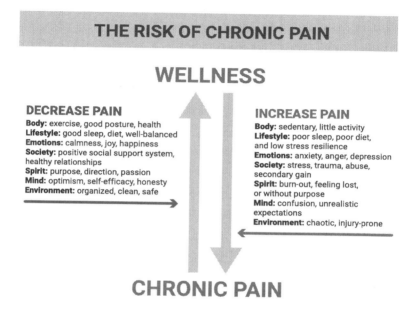

THE RISK OF CHRONIC PAIN

WELLNESS

DECREASE PAIN
Body: exercise, good posture, health
Lifestyle: good sleep, diet, well-balanced
Emotions: calmness, joy, happiness
Society: positive social support system, healthy relationships
Spirit: purpose, direction, passion
Mind: optimism, self-efficacy, honesty
Environment: organized, clean, safe

INCREASE PAIN
Body: sedentary, little activity
Lifestyle: poor sleep, poor diet, and low stress resilience
Emotions: anxiety, anger, depression
Society: stress, trauma, abuse, secondary gain
Spirit: burn-out, feeling lost, or without purpose
Mind: confusion, unrealistic expectations
Environment: chaotic, injury-prone

CHRONIC PAIN

Adapted from *Practical Pain Management* (Friction et. al)

Pain Habit #1 - Poor Posture

Certain body parts, much like certain people, become habituated to pain more easily than others. We see this especially with neck and shoulder pain, as well as low back and hip pain, which are often caused by habitually poor posture. This is a significant issue because people sit too much and too often employ poor posture. The American Medical Association (AMA) recently publicized a new slogan - 'Sitting is the new smoking' - to raise awareness and help people understand how this epidemic is affecting their health.

In support of this, Harvard University published a study demonstrating that when you improve your posture, you increase your self-confidence, reduce depression and anxiety, as well as improve digestion, blood flow, and oxygen to the brain and body. The study also showed that, by sitting and standing in an upright posture, aging can be reversed, and life expectancy can increase.

Unfortunately, while it's all too clear how much sitting negatively impacts the body, so many of today's jobs are sedentary. Sitting results in shortened muscles, tight joints, fascial restrictions, and strained ligaments. Your spinal joints, called 'facet joints,' are loaded with special receptors or sensors that bombard the brain with pain messages when you slump and have poor posture. No wonder so many people suffer from pain in the low back and neck. Below is a diagram depicting the most common postures. Poor postures are depicted on the left and in the middle. Optimal ones are displayed on the right.

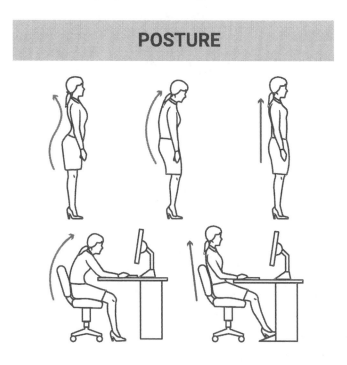

Posture Hacks

To optimize posture and reduce pain, research shows that there are different types of physical therapy that work best. When you're having pain, serial deep tissue massage twice a week can help to calm the overly-excited receptors in your joints that bombard the nervous system. Over time, this gradually reduces chemical inflammation and decreases pain. The most effective type of physical therapy does require your active participation. By moving your affected body parts against some manual resistance, you can inhibit pain and enhance range of motion. This is an active form of therapy and can be experienced in Muscle Energy Techniques (MET), Active Release Therapy (ART), Muscle Activation Therapy (MAT), and active dry needling. If you are interested in finding a therapist or provider in your area I encourage you to do some research online or ask friends, family or medical providers for their recommendations. Other considerations to improve your posture include:

- Change your routine. Avoid doing the same activities or exercises every day.
- Change your shoes often and wear different heel types.
- Avoid carrying heavy things on the same side of your body.
- Become aware of your dominant standing leg and avoid leaning on it while standing for long periods.
- Breathe diaphragmatically and engage your core.
- Spread your stance and take up space.
- Use a sit/stand desk and set a timer to remind you to get up frequently and change position.
- If you have poor body awareness, consider using posture biofeedback devices to remind you of when you're slouching.

- Avoid sitting on couches that are overly soft and non-supportive of neutral postures.
- Adjust your car seat to optimize your sitting angle and minimize strain on your hamstrings and arms.
- Avoid looking down at books, cell phones, tablets, and other electronic devices for long periods of time.
- Avoid sitting with your legs tightly crossed, because it positions your pelvis in a twisted posture and reduces circulation of blood to your legs.

Pain Habit #2 - Poor Body Awareness

Another feature of poor posture is poor body awareness. Unfortunately, many of us have never learned good body awareness. Body awareness begins as early in life as four to six months and it's something that we must practice to become good at. When people have trauma, surgery, or challenging childhoods, they often miss out on the optimal neurodevelopmental stages that lead to body awareness. If this sounds like you, then you may be more likely to have poor posture and pain later in life. If you are someone who has never challenged your body to perform at peak levels, it may be that your body awareness has never been fully developed. As the saying goes, if you don't use it, you lose it.

Body awareness is important because it informs you where your body is in the space around you. It's similar to your other senses, clueing you in on the state of affairs in the body. This happens as your brain forms 'maps' which carry information about all of your body parts and how they relate to one another. People with poor body awareness often refer to themselves as clumsy, klutzy, and uncoordinated. They have a hard time developing muscle memory in sports and they may have difficulty with fine motor coordination and developing automatic movements.

Until one learns how to become aware of their body, it's hard to learn new motor skills. That's why it's difficult for some people to learn a new sport as they get older. Body awareness involves the coordination of the brain and body and strongly impacts one's sense of self. In tests where people with poor body awareness were asked to draw a self-portrait, they often depicted body parts out of proportion. Some even had missing body parts.

Body awareness and posture work hand in glove. There are wonderful ways to improve body awareness at any age. Dancing is helpful, pilates and yoga are also beneficial. Conscious breathing and body scan meditations are immensely helpful and can be done for free at home. These practices help to facilitate body awareness and calm the stress/ threat response by stimulating the vagus nerve. Additional information about these techniques will be presented in later chapters. When you give your brain and nervous system something to do, it forces your brain to pay attention to those parts of the body, eventually helping empower you to change old habits.

Additional things you can do to improve body awareness include:

- Standing and balancing on a Bosu ball or uneven surface.
- Hopping on one leg.
- Jumping rope.
- Playing games that involve naming and drawing body parts.
- Mirror games.
- Use of obstacle courses to improve agility.
- Use of a rebounder or mini trampoline.

Body Awareness and Nonjudgmental Self-Acceptance

Nonjudgmental self-acceptance of your body is an important feature of self-awareness. This means that you unconditionally love and accept yourself for who you really are, including those things you like about yourself and those that you don't. Nonjudgmental self-acceptance is an active process, rather than a passive one, requiring a willingness to fully experience your thoughts, feelings, and emotions without denial.

Some people have difficulty accepting this concept because we are taught at an early age to compare ourselves to the images of models and movie stars, which few of us can measure up to. When we see past the unrealistic marketing influences that bombard us across all forms of media, as well as the relentless social pressures to conform, we can begin to accept who we are: warts and all. We can then start to embrace nonjudgmental self-acceptance and learn to appreciate our bodies for the marvels that they are, accepting ourselves in the process.

This is one of the first steps to self-acceptance and self-love, helping us to develop self-confidence, improve our social skills, and build emotional intelligence. As you become more aware of your body in space, you start to pay more attention to your body language and the signals you send out to others. You also begin to draw realistic associations between how you feel and how you think.

For example, when you feel nervous and have a queasy feeling in your stomach, your heart rate increases, and your face gets flushed. This is how you can begin to understand how your emotions and stress affect your physiology and biochemistry. With practice, you can start to sense even the slightest effects and take corrective action to bring your emotions and physiology back into balance. When your self-awareness is intact, you can more easily and consciously move into an optimal state of inner and outer balance (homeostasis). This phenomenon is the state of perfect balance between your thoughts, feelings, and emotions, and the effects they have on your body.

Body Awareness and Stress

In the earlier chapters, you explored how pain and stress are flip sides of the same coin. You also learned that by changing the way you mentally perceive pain, you can profoundly alter how you experience pain on a physiological level. A major advantage of improving body awareness is that, as you practice it, you become more likely to notice the early effects that stress, anxiety, and tension have on you. When your body awareness is intact, it becomes a reliable indicator of whether you've overdone it and need to take a break.

Without this valuable feedback mechanism to tell you that you're out of balance, you often ignore the important messages that your body is trying to send. Further, when you suppress these early warning signs and neglect your basic needs for proper nutrition, adequate hydration, digestion, and rest, you will face negative consequences of pain and 'dis-ease.' With practice, as you improve your body awareness, you'll understand more readily what the body really needs. For example, you'll be more likely to notice if you eat something or do something that doesn't agree with you. Irregular bowel habits, gassiness, and bloating, may lead you to explore the possibility of food intolerances, such as gluten, dairy, corn, peanuts, eggs, and others. If you're experiencing back and neck strain, you might conclude that you are sitting for too long in an unsupported posture or using a chair that lacks proper support.

Pain Habit #3 - Poor Breathing Patterns

It may come as a surprise, but most people breathe improperly. Unfortunately, poor breathing habits can make you sick and cause pain. Why? Since many people go through their day with a substantial amount of stress hormones circulating in their bloodstream and their autonomic nervous system is geared for fight or flight, their breathing patterns reflect this. This is because breathing is a function of our autonomic nervous system.

Some common dysfunctional breathing patterns include: rapid shallow breathing, chest breathing, mouth breathing, sighing, yawning, and breath holding. Reverse breathing is also a common dysfunctional pattern. This occurs when the diaphragm pulls up into the chest with inhalation and drops into the abdomen during exhalation. Reverse breathing is the opposite of normal breathing, which is characterized by the diaphragm moving down with inhalation and moving up with exhalation. One thing that is commonly associated with poor breathing habits is lack of awareness of how we breathe along with poor body awareness. Improvement in both of these areas is important because proper breathing serves to purify our blood, remove toxins, improve our brain, sexual, and GI function, and massage the internal organs. The beneficial effects of improving breathing patterns are often immediate.

Another surprising fact about breathing is that many people are unaware of how many muscles are involved in the process. Optimal breathing involves the coordinated movement of the diaphragm, intercostal chest wall muscles, abdominal muscles, back muscles (quadratus lumborum), pectoralis muscles, and two neck muscles (the sternocleidomastoids and the scalenes). Unfortunately, most people don't use the most important breathing muscle - their diaphragm - and instead rely too heavily on their

79

accessory or emergency muscles to breathe. This makes breathing an inefficient process, causing additional stress on the system, creating and reinforcing poor postural patterns such as 'forward head', tight pectorals, high-riding rib cage, and lack of core muscle engagement.

The Breathing Retraining Center has identified healthy breathing habits that I would like to share with you.

- Breathe through your nose all the time even when eating, speaking, and exercising.
- Be mindful of an upright posture when sitting or standing to optimize your air flow.
- Breathe into your diaphragm - belly breathing rather than chest breathing improves health.
- Breathe in a regular pattern in terms of rate and depth of each breath.
- Breathe 8 - 12 breaths per minute.
- Match your breathing to your activity and then make sure to cool down the breath as you would any muscle after exercise.
- Allow breathing to happen without expending too much energy.
- Practice relaxation of muscles and thoughts. Select positive thoughts and feelings as much as possible, because it affects how much air you need.
- Slowly master breath hold time after you master all other habits.
- Strengthen your diaphragm with exercises such as laying on your back with your knees bent and place a book on top of your belly. Then practice breathing into your belly so that the book moves up and then down. Breathing while

standing in water up to your chest or swimming using a snorkel is also helpful to strengthen the diaphragm, as you have the added resistance of the water to push against.

Some recommend a breathing exercise called 'the lifter,' that you do only once a day. The steps are as follows:

- Stand with your upper body supported on your knees.
- Take at least three deep breaths to prepare yourself.
- When you feel that you have oxygenated sufficiently, blow all of your air out, hold your breath, and then suck in your lower belly tight against your spine.
- Hold the position and your breath for several seconds or for as long as you can.
- Relax the belly before breathing again.
- Repeat at least three times or until you are exhausted.

Alternate nostril breathing is another breathing exercise that is helpful to improve breath awareness and deep breathing, while also stimulating the parasympathetic nervous system and activating the Vagus Nerve to calm us down. In yoga circles, this is called Nadi Shodhana. Here's how it works. Hold your left nostril closed using your right pinky finger, exhale once, and then inhale once through the right nostril. Then, close the right nostril using the thumb of your right hand, exhale once and inhale once through the left nostril. Continue switching from side to side for 9 breaths on each side. At the completion of each round of nine breaths take 3 resting breaths through both nostrils.

Pain Habit #4 - Lack of Grounding

Your body is a vastly interconnected system with your feet as the foundation. Being well-grounded means that you are aware of your feet on the ground and you are connected to the earth's electromagnetic field. When you are linked to the earth in this way, you are more likely to be attuned to environmental cues. It's no different than any other electrical device that has to be grounded to the earth's electromagnetic field to work. Being grounded is a significant determinant in health because your cells transmit electrical frequencies that operate your heart, muscles, nervous system, and immune function. People who are well grounded are more centered, more balanced, and less tense. They have decreased levels of stress, inflammation, and pain, and report improved sleep.

On the other hand, when you are ungrounded, living in chronic pain and under constant stress, you will likely suffer fatigue, anxiety, or depression. When you go to seek medical advice, it may not be easy to find the cause of your suffering. This is when practitioners resort to prescribing medications to manage symptoms. The unfortunate truth is that many, if not all, of these drugs have side effects that exacerbate fatigue and cause GI issues, constipation, and foggy thinking. In my experience, being ungrounded is a significant risk factor for opioid dependence.

I ask every patient who comes to see me to take off their shoes and walk down the hall. This gives me a chance to see how well-grounded they are and allows me to assess their 'centeredness' and body awareness. What I tell my patients is that your feet are where your back meets the ground. I find it interesting how few people today pay attention to the feet, which determine one's 'stance' in life, providing stability and firm roots. One simple exercise I suggest to my patients is the short foot exercise, which helps wake up the muscles in your feet and strengthen them. This exercise involves standing and contracting the arch of your foot, effectively making your footprint shorter and your arch higher. Hold the contraction of your foot muscles for ten seconds, then release and repeat.

There are 26 foot bones and over 100 muscles, tendons, and ligaments in the feet. These structures help you absorb shock, deal with gravity, propel you through space, and provide valuable sensory input to your brain. For athletes, strengthening one's feet has very positive effects on their performance. A recent study in the Journal of Physical Therapy Science showed that simple foot strengthening exercises can improve strength, running speed, and horizontal and vertical jump distance. This would translate to enhanced performance on the golf course and tennis court as well. Any standing sport from skiing to surfing involves our feet, so investing time on strengthening the feet will pay big dividends.

Whether you're an athlete or not, your body is the great master of compensation. For example, when your feet function poorly, your other tissues have to pick up the slack. This phenomenon is called the 'kinetic chain.' To be more light-hearted, this is another way of saying that the foot bone is connected to the knee bone and the knee bone is connected to the hip bone. Your fascia is the flat elastic tissue that separates your muscles, connecting your entire body from head to toe. When key muscles, such as those in your feet, are weak, you will automatically overuse other muscles, causing overuse syndromes that lead to pain.

Exercises to improve foot function:

- Short foot exercise or standing on the ball mounts of your feet and lifting up your toes. This is an element of many standing poses in yoga.
- Going barefoot or wearing minimalist shoes help our feet get grounded. Walking barefoot on the beach.
- Rolling a ball under your foot to release tendons, muscles, and the plantar fascia. You can use a lacrosse ball or

tennis ball to do this. Small round frozen water bottles are also helpful tools to roll out tension in your feet. It's also possible to mobilize stiff joints in your feet using this technique.

- Standing and walking on your heels and toes.
- Kneeling with your toes tucked under yourself and crawling on all fours. This stretches and strengthens your foot muscles and helps to improve your coordination and activates your core.
- Mobilizing your big toe is also helpful, because it's the first and most crucial joint in the gait sequence. Every step begins with bending the big toe. If that joint is stiff, then you will surely have compensation patterns all the way up the kinetic chain.

Pain Habit #5 - Poor Sleep Hygiene

Our lives revolve around two states: arousal (when you're awake) and sleep. To be sure, sleep is a critical component in the process of maintaining homeostasis. When we don't sleep well, we move into a state of fatigue and exhaustion that cause stress. Pain can cause sleep deprivation by impeding the sleep drive. Studies show that people with chronic pain that is accompanied by insomnia, have higher levels of disability. Moreover, people with chronic pain and depression have more significant sleep disorders. Sleep is one of our most important daily habits. Your behaviors during the day, and especially at night, have a significant impact on your sleep.

Some poor sleep habits include:

- Going to bed at inconsistent times.
- Getting less than seven hours of sleep.

- Waiting until you are sleepy to go to bed.
- Getting out of bed when you can't fall asleep.
- Being exposed to light, media, and mental stimulation before bed.
- Drinking alcohol, caffeine, and excessive fluids before bed.
- Sleeping in a recliner chair, rather than in a bed.

Many of my patients tell me that the only way they can get comfortable at night is in a recliner chair. It would be negligent if I didn't explain how sleeping in a recliner chair can be just as bad for you as sitting for long periods. It leads to shortening and contractures of your hip flexors and hamstrings, which are the muscles that control your upright posture. When these muscles are tight, they affect your balance and distort your posture.

We all have individual preferences in our sleep posture. Some prefer lying on their back, while others prefer lying on their side in a 'fetal' position. Sleeping in a bed allows you to relax your body in a horizontal position, reducing pressure on the spine, and allowing fluids to rehydrate our discs while we sleep. Sleeping in a recliner may be okay for short periods of time, such as post-surgery, during bouts of breathing distress or the final weeks of pregnancy, as well as because of sleep apnea, congestive heart failure, or severe heartburn. However, making this a long-term habit is not advisable.

There are, of course, many reasons why people don't sleep well. In Chapter 8, which explores 'Health as a Habit,' I review some additional recommendations for establishing good sleep hygiene.

Pain Habit #6 - Poor Nutrition

For many of us, our eating habits are often hard to change. Many people do not know what good nutrition really looks like. In recent years we have discovered that what we eat affects how we feel. Researchers from the University of Alabama discovered that chronic pain patients who have poor diets are more prone to suffer excessive pain and develop other chronic diseases.

To be clear, it's not just about weight gain. Our food can either reduce inflammation or create it, leading to insulin resistance (sometimes called pre-diabetes). Poor nutrition can disrupt normal recovery from injuries and exaggerate pain levels. The most problematic addictive substances are sugar, caffeine, and alcohol. These substances are known to increase cortisol levels, which creates negative ripple effects leading to inflammation. Other nutrition habits that contribute to pain include skipping meals, eating excessive portions, and eating the same things every day.

Two of the most important daily habits that I discuss with all of my patients are their diet and bowel habits. Identifying a potential "gut-brain-pain connection" in each patient is important, given that inflammation often starts in the gut. Of course, many people manage stress by consuming (or over-consuming) sugar, caffeine, and alcohol. The resulting escalation of cortisol primes the body for pain and poor health. A hidden source of sugar is high fructose corn syrup, which is cheaper and sweeter than real sugar, it's frequently a main ingredient in condiments, such as ketchup and store bought salad dressings. The problem with high fructose corn syrup is that it is highly processed, poorly digested, and is not absorbed by the body. Dr. Mark Hyman argues that it is better to eat foods with small amounts of natural sugar than to consume any amount of high fructose corn syrup. Other common food issues include eating pro-inflammatory foods such as processed or pre-prepared foods, trans fats, as well as gluten and dairy. Nightshade vegetables such as peppers, tomatoes, potatoes and eggplant can also cause inflammation in some people. In Chapter 8, I will address healthy nutrition habits in greater detail.

Pain Habit #7 - Perfectionism

Pain and perfectionism, in many ways, are the perfect pair. Dr. John Sarno was one of the most prominent proponents of perfectionism as a cause of chronic pain. He described people with perfectionistic personalities as the ultimate people pleasers. While they strive to make others happy, they often don't practice unconditional self-love and self-acceptance. Perfectionism often starts in childhood. Strict upbringings often lead perfectionists to consciously or unconsciously believe they are not good enough. As a result, they expend tremendous amounts of energy trying to perfect their behavior.

Because perfectionists are constantly gauging their self-worth by how they're perceived by other people, they lose their own internal compass for self-awareness. In turn, this impacts their authentic self-confidence. Without external feedback from others, perfectionists really don't know who they are. It was Dr. Sarno's belief that even though perfectionists consciously embrace their 'do-gooder nature,' their mind is busy subconsciously harboring deep resentment over the pain of 'not being good enough.' Maintaining this internal emotional conflict takes its toll over time. These deep wounds bubble up, and must eventually come into the light of conscious awareness. It was Dr. Sarno's belief that knowing how this happens in our subconscious mind empowers us to be able to choose consciously to process these feelings and release them.

Scientists from Northwestern University have shown that, in the mind, "state-dependent learning renders stressful fear-related memories consciously inaccessible." This means that we are wired such that our memories are most accessible when we are in the same state of consciousness as we were when the memory was formed. Dr. Sarno recognized that state-dependent learning allows our subconscious mind to shield our conscious mind from traumatic memories. This explains yet another reason that Post-Traumatic Stress Disorder (PTSD) is so hard to treat. Moreover, they also shield us from bringing the emotional trauma associated with maintaining a perfectionistic personality into our full awareness. It was Sarno's belief that, in order to protect these subconscious emotional wounds, our mind creates pain as a conscious distraction. Furthermore, health coach Anhaita Parseghian argues that "anyone who has experienced chronic pain knows that it dominates and consumes one's entire life and mind, leaving little emotional or physical bandwidth, making pain perhaps the most effective defense mechanism against bringing subconscious thoughts into awareness."

However, by becoming aware of this subconscious process, we can break through and begin to disable the defense mechanisms at the root of the pain and suffering. Like in the Wizard of Oz, as we pull back the curtain, becoming aware of what was previously just a belief stuck in our subconscious, our pain loses its power over us, often disappearing. As such, the ultimate keys to outsmarting our pain lie in our understanding of how the mind works and how we can learn to adapt in life more effectively.

All-or-Nothing Thinking

Dr. Murray McAllister published a fantastic summary of perfectionism and chronic pain in the May 2015 edition for The Institute for Chronic Pain. Dr. McAllister describes another aspect of perfectionism that leads to chronic pain: 'all-or-nothing' thinking. This has what he describes as a "boom-and-bust effect in their lives, because they're either too busy pushing their limits to the breaking point, or they just give up and do nothing." In other words, there's never a happy medium, nor is there any consideration that pacing oneself is even an option.

Fear of Failure and Fear of the Unknown

Dr. McAllister argues that "perfectionists cannot accept failure and they do everything in their power to avoid it. Paralyzed by the fear of getting it wrong, they instead do nothing. They would rather risk inaction than put themselves in a position of possible failure." When we're fearful of what the future holds, we're trapped in our mind. When fear takes hold of us, we often sit and mull over our various options, rather than be proactive and take the steps to move forward. Because of their need for perfection, these people don't want to make a bad decision. Because they simply don't trust themselves, they take forever to make a choice. They process everything mentally, failing to trust their intuition or 'felt sense.'

Pacing

For the perfectionist, pacing is an enigma. The compulsive need to stay busy and get the job done right comes with the cost of exacerbating pain. Learning to pace oneself requires accepting that we need to find a middle ground between these two extremes. Perfectionists struggle with the notion that things in their life can be 'just good enough' and have that be an agreeable outcome.

Because of this inherent challenge, when perfectionists develop chronic pain, it can be difficult to treat. The real focus of treating perfectionists with chronic pain should revolve around improving their self-awareness and expanding their insight. This helps them see what's really working in their lives, and what's working against them, weakening their defenses, and causing pain and 'dis-ease.'

In almost everything they do, perfectionists have a sense of urgency to meet unattainably high standards. This compulsion creates all kinds of tension, which is also perpetuated by the persistent negative emotional states that form the core operating system of the inner life of a perfectionist. Perfectionists often feel unsatisfied with life, and as a result, they find it hard to fully relax. A genuine sense of inner peace always remains just outside of their reach.

Perfectionism and Opioids

Some perfectionists try to solve their all-or-nothing dilemma by relying on pain-relieving drugs called opioids. The downside is that these drugs are highly addictive and aren't genuine long-term solutions to pain. Opioids certainly reduce the symptoms of pain, but in doing so, they give the perfectionist a false sense of feeling good, promoting their agenda of going 'all in.' They pursue perfect, superhuman feats, and when they fall short, they suffer much more. This is the start of the cycle of drug dependency. Clearly, using opioids to medicate behaviorally-exacerbated pain is not ideal. It would be healthier and more effective for them to learn to overcome perfectionism and develop self-awareness and effective pacing skills.

Pain Habit #8 - Overthinking Pain

Some people are worrywarts and that's all there is to it. People who dwell on the negative experience of pain are called 'catastrophizers.' They ruminate over their pain. This is a cognitive distortion involving unhelpful and/or unrealistic beliefs about pain. Many, if not all of us, have heard their tales of woe and stories of victimhood.

Catastrophizing is such an important risk factor for chronic pain that the 'Pain Catastrophizing Scale' was established by Dr. Michael Sullivan of McGill University. In his User Manual he describes three distinct facets. First, the exaggeration of the threat value of pain (pain magnification). Second, perseverative thinking about pain (rumination). Third, underestimation of one's coping ability (Learned Helplessness Scale).

It's important to understand that it's not just about our thoughts, but rather the beliefs we hold about our thoughts that determine how much attention we give them. Overanalyzing or 'analysis paralysis' is counterproductive because it causes you to dwell on the problem rather than the solution.

Overthinking keeps us mentally circling between the past and the future, so that our present goes on without us. When we develop mental loops about pain, our most creative solutions become inaccessible to us. Another troubling aspect lies in the fact that people who live in the past are prone to depression and people who live in the future are prone to anxiety.

The irony is that, when you focus your energy on worrying about pain, you're likely to experience more of it. When our mind is confused, and we feel anxious, we eventually experience physical symptoms in the form of pain and fatigue. When physical issues are caused by stress from our disordered mental loops, it doesn't mean the problem is all in our heads. Rather, it's the embodied stress response that causes the pain.

People who overthink their pain are plagued by distressing thoughts. Their inability to get out of their own heads leaves them in a state of constant emotional anguish, making it hard for them to connect with other people. This persistent emotional distress leads many overthinkers to resort to unhealthy coping strategies, such as abusing drugs, alcohol, food, and developing toxic relationships. All of these behaviors contribute to prolonging, or even intensifying, pain.

Physical manifestations of overthinking and perfectionism include:

- Frequent headaches
- Mental exhaustion
- Fatigue from overdoing
- Stiff muscles and joints

Overthinking starts in the mind, but it creeps into other parts of the body leaving you feeling tight, tired, and fatigued. Once emotions get involved, we tend to hold onto discomfort until the underlying emotional issue gets resolved.

Like perfectionism, overthinking is a dysfunctional behavioral pattern that leads to pain. If you're a person with these patterns, you would be well-served by an educational program designed to help you cultivate a more positive relationship with yourself, focused on teaching new approaches for managing your thoughts and emotions. This would be far more beneficial than taking habit-forming medications. This way your thoughts and emotions become friendly guideposts on your journey through life.

Ways to avoid overthinking and catastrophizing pain include:

- Increase your self-awareness. Notice when you think too much and associate your thoughts with how you feel.
- Don't believe everything you think. Challenge your thoughts, especially negative ones about pain.
- Focus on the solution to your pain and not the pain problem. This helps you gain access to higher-level thinking and more creative solutions.
- Find small actions you can take to alleviate pain and track your progress.
- Schedule time for reflection and relaxation. Set a timer for ten to twenty minutes and try to do so multiple times throughout the day.
- Practice mindfulness and awareness of the present moment. Consider using the body scan meditation, because it helps to takes you out of your head and back into your body.
- Release fear of the unknown and the need to control everything.
- Make sure you turn your mind off at night, so that you get restful sleep. The mind is like a computer that needs to shut down completely, so that it can refresh itself.
- Consider professional counseling with a therapist or life coach skilled in techniques such as cognitive-behavioral therapy, acceptance and commitment therapy, and mindfulness.

Reasons why we feel stuck in pain:

- Doing the same things in terms of thinking or emotional patterns, while expecting a different response.
- Lack of body awareness and proper exercise sequencing
- Constant worrying
- Unproductive habits
- Constant disappointment and feeling like a victim
- Limited hope for the future
- Unclear goals and lack of focus
- Not having enough energy, because of physical and mental drain
- Lack of self-confidence
- Lack of inspiration
- Unwillingness to take self-responsibility
- Lack of information
- Lack of a clear plan

Unfortunately, it's all too easy to fall into a painful rut, something which all people have experienced in their lives. When we get stuck in pain, we tend to wait for external factors to shift. However, meaningful changes don't typically happen to us; they originate from within us. You must believe that you have the power to make the essential changes in how you think, act, and view your circumstances. This makes you a powerful creator of your own reality, because each of us is fully responsible for what happens in our lives.

A helpful way of releasing the grip of pain is to first acknowledge what needs to change, then let go of past hurts and disappointments. This process of release often involves forgiving yourself and others, setting yourself free from painful memories, and telling different stories. When you believe in yourself, you learn to trust in your inner guidance, knowing that it will show you a better way. This allows you access to your instincts and intuition, helping you to make your best decisions. Deciding to move beyond pain is an emotional process that requires courage, self-love, and commitment. Moreover, it requires you to recognize life's challenges as opportunities for growth.

Yoga teaches us that 'the body's truth goes ahead of the mind's lie.' Our bodies are designed to provide us with access to a special kind of physiologic wisdom that bypasses the mind. When we make decisions purely based on our intellect, without listening to the deeper 'body truth,' we may miss out on important messages and signposts along the way. Looking at it another way, pain and misery may be 'life' asking you to become a better listener, so that your choices become more heartfelt and authentic, and based less on mental habits and past conditioning.

There are many helpful tools you can use to get unstuck, including tracking progress through charting and journaling. Many people like using habit or routine tracking applications like *Way of Life, Habitica,* or *HabitBull* to monitor their efforts and progress toward a goal. These have been shown to be very helpful in facilitating behavior change. Each app offers slightly different approaches, so you may need to experiment to find the one best suited for you.

Breaking the pain habit means different things to each of us. If you recognize yourself being described, I hope this book gives you valuable information and useful tools to help you increase your self-awareness and overcome your pain.

It's amazing when we stop to think of the total impact of pain. So many people in the world suffer with chronic pain, without knowing why. I'm hopeful that in learning how pain can become a habit, you can consciously choose to change it. When you opt to not make deliberate choices, you fall back on whatever feels natural or most comfortable, such as your previous pain-perpetuating habits. Remember, outsmarting your pain rarely takes you down the path of least resistance.

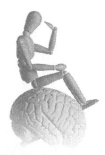

Chapter 5

Know Your Pain Triggers

"Your body never lies. It says what words cannot."

- Martha Graham

Exploring Your Pain and Stress Triggers

We are feeling, sensing, and thinking organisms. When you consider your pain triggers, you have to look at your internal thoughts and emotions, as well as your external environmental exposures. According to psychologist Dr. Margaret Paul, one of the reasons we all have triggers is because of our experiences as children. She explains that, "When we were growing up, we inevitably experienced pain or suffering that we could not acknowledge and/or deal with sufficiently at that time. So, as adults, we typically become triggered by experiences that are reminiscent of the really old painful feelings." These ideas are supported by the work of Dr. Stephen Porges, author of *The Polyvagal Theory,* who asks the question - are we are all traumatized in some way?

These triggers don't even have to be particularly traumatic. All that's required is that they have been persistent enough to cause you distress. As a result of this, we typically turn to a habitual or addictive way of trying to manage painful feelings. Healing childhood wounds - what some call the inner child - is important to stop the pain triggers. Therapy or coaching is helpful in rooting these childhood patterns out. If you avoid dealing with these old wounds, you will stay stuck in a pattern of self-defeating behaviors.

Trauma itself can also be a pain trigger and it's typically a deeply distressing experience. At the moment of trauma, we take mental and emotional snapshots of the event, causing us to continually relive the negative experience in the future. Because of the mental and visual 'pictures' we take at the time of the trauma, we develop mental loops to the experience. Therapies such as 'Eye Movement Desensitization Retraining' (EMDR) and 'Brain-spotting' are very helpful in breaking these patterns. I have also found hypnotherapy to be helpful for some of my patients suffering from post-traumatic stress disorder (PTSD) as it is a 'back-door' approach to addressing hidden issues stored in the subconscious mind. Neurofeedback is also an effective modality to help with PTSD as it helps to rewire neural pathways. The device monitors your brainwaves and rewards you when you are in an 'optimal' mental state.

According to neuroscientist Antonio Damasio, "feelings are mental experiences of body states." Damasio asserts that, "emotions play out in the theatre of the body" while "feelings play out in the theatre of the mind." The word 'emotion' comes from the Latin word 'emovere,' which means 'to set in motion.' Remember that your emotions can set in motion a cascade of physiological effects that play out in our bodies in various ways, which is the basis of the concept of psychoneuroimmunology.

Your body recognizes negative emotions by how it responds - trembling with fear, crying with grief, and convulsing with anger and disgust. The important thing to remember is to ask your body questions. Why do I hurt? What is my body trying to tell me? What do I need to embrace? What do I need to let go of? You might be surprised by the answers.

Scientists have confirmed the mind-body connection by mapping out the effects of different emotional states on our bodily sensations. Studies conducted in Sweden, Finland, and Taiwan came to some consistent conclusions. Sensations in the arms were closely associated with the emotions of anger and happiness. Leg sensations were connected with sadness. Sensations in the abdomen and throat were linked to the emotion of disgust.

Sometimes emotions are triggered by your thoughts. Remember that your thoughts are just thoughts and they may be inaccurate. Feeling something doesn't make it true. This is where your old patterns can trip you up, because every time you react to a thought, belief, or an emotion, you make it harder not to react the next time.

Many of us adopt painful limiting beliefs as 'our story.' Once you tell your story, you feel justified in carrying on certain self-destructive behaviors that go along with it. When we stay stuck in our story, we continually repeat the same experiences.

In Chapter 1, you explored the involvement of the autonomic nervous system (ANS) to your thoughts, feelings, and emotions. Neuroscientist Candace Pert, in her book, *Your Body is Your Subconscious Mind*, argues that your body always perfectly mirrors your subconscious mind. In turn, your internal story, which you tell yourself and your body, speaks to you through emotions, which communicate through your autonomic nervous system directly to your cells.

Positive and Negative Emotions

We all have positive and negative emotions; both being part of the richness of life. Emotional intelligence is actually 'body intelligence,' which refers to our body's ability to feel our emotions fully. However, some of us are completely emotion-phobic. Emotion phobia dissociates us from the trapped energy residue in our muscles, signaling to us that these emotions are scary and destructive. When this happens, we see them as a threat, which generates the threat response.

Every 'dark' or negative emotion has value in teaching us important life lessons. For example, psychotherapist Miriam Greenspan states that grief teaches that "we are interconnected with the web of life, and that what connects us also breaks our hearts." When you experience grief, do your best to be mindful about it. Sit with it and let it wash over you. Befriend it and let it be. Three emotional skills you can refine to help you deal with challenging thoughts and emotions are: attending to them, befriending them, and surrendering to them. This is similar to what is taught in the RAIN method discussed in Chapter 4.

Miriam Greenspan also asserts that negative emotions - like fear, grief, and despair - are as much a part of the human condition as positive emotions, such as love, awe, and joy. Many people try to live in a culture of positivity, with an overriding bias toward positive emotions of joy, love, pride, compassion, hope, and happiness. However, negative emotions are an important part of life too. Research is now revealing that experiencing and accepting difficult emotions is vital to our resilience and mental health. As you will soon explore, learning to identify them, name them, and tame them, will help you to disarm them from triggering your threat response.

Negative emotions most connected with a heightened threat response are:

- Fear
- Sadness
- Anger
- Shame
- Grief
- Despair
- Envy
- Jealousy
- Guilt
- Rage
- Surprise
- Disgust
- Contempt

Cut Shame Out of the Game

It's not uncommon for us to hide our emotional triggers, because we don't want to seem vulnerable or look weak. Author and professor Brene Brown points out that, when we feel negative emotions, we sometimes feel 'flawed.' Shame is that painful emotion associated with the sense of feeling like a failure. Unlike guilt, which is a negative emotion associated with our behavior, shame is an emotion that defines us. Maybe we let someone we care about down, or we fell short of achieving a personal goal we set for ourselves. Either way, we don't feel worthy enough. Shame is the embodiment of self-judgement. Shame robs us of the possibility of experiencing joy, leaving our positive feelings interrupted, and our life on permanent hold. But, what does shame 'feel' like? Physical reactions to shame include: flushing of the face and neck, sweating, a sunken chest, and bowing our heads down. We hold ourselves in guarded postures.

'Toxic shame' is a term coined by psychotherapist Silvan Tomkins. He says, "unlike normal shame, toxic shame stays buried within your mind, ultimately becoming part of your self-identity, leading to low self-esteem and self-loathing." Even when we feel shame about something trivial, it often makes us feel like we want to hide.

Shame is so pervasive and daunting, but it doesn't have a tangible location in our 'mental space'. It's like wearing emotional camouflage. When we are angry, sad, jealous, or feel guilty, we can usually easily identify these emotions. Shame is different. When we have shame from painful past experiences, such as abuse, abandonment, or neglect it's like a 'circuit breaker' that can disrupt your sense of self worth and trigger your nervous system to feel a potential threat. However, you don't usually know why. Many chronic pain sufferers have this theme running in the background of their lives, quietly derailing their health. To make matters worse, people who feel 'shamed' often unknowingly project blame and anger on others. The shamed person wants to regain some semblance of control and power yet this behavior pushes people away causing isolation and loneliness.

For all of the reasons we have identified, and more, there's no doubt that shame is prevalent in our culture. I encourage you to read Brené Brown's book, *Daring Greatly*, and learn how to work with the emotion of shame, so that it doesn't trigger your pain. In the book, she teaches Shame Resilience, a four step process to learn how to effectively express your emotions, without attachment or judgement. It gives you the freedom to allow your emotions to take leave of your body and liberates you from the extra baggage you carry around in your muscles. As you feel your way through this negative emotion, you figure out what messages and expectations trigger it.

Remember that most of our emotional triggers stem from not having our needs met. Our emotional needs include the need for love, acceptance, safety, fun, peacefulness, autonomy, and respect, as well as being treated fairly, feeling valued, and having a sense of control over our circumstances. It's helpful to reflect on what unmet needs or desires you may have.

Now that you better understand the mind-body connection, you know that you can't divorce your health from your emotions. According to health coach K.G. Stiles, "Your emotions are invisible energies in motion that move through you with lightning-fast speed, flooding you with signals of either pleasure or pain. Like brush strokes on a blank canvas, your emotions color your world with contrast and meaning." Every emotion is felt somewhere in the body. When we are stressed out and not taking care of ourselves, the painful effects are even more severe. Remember that many of us don't always know us how and where our emotions affect us. We just need to more fully observe how we physically feel.

Self-Destructive vs. Self-Supportive Behaviors

In general, there are two kinds of mindsets: self-destructive and self-supportive. The feeling state of a self-destructive person is fear. With this mindset, one allows fear to have the power to influence their behavior. They learn at an early age to forfeit their responsibility for how they feel, allowing other people to have that control. Additionally, self-destructive behaviors can provide relief from pain and even stimulate pleasure in the moment. However, in the long run, they create problems for those seeking a truly fulfilling life.

Self-destructive or 'dysregulated' behaviors start early in life and are often a response to adverse childhood events. The behaviors are often associated with denial of negative emotions that seem too much to bear. The self destructive person never really processes their emotions. They just stay there like a pot on the stove. Imagine putting an air-tight lid on a pot of boiling water; the boiling water and the steam are still there. Self-destructive behaviors can, and often do, become painful habits. The key to breaking those habits is to get in touch with the underlying emotional triggers.

But that means you must face your emotions, sooner or later. Seeking help from a compassionate friend, health coach, or therapist will be very helpful in breaking self-destructive emotional and behavioral habits. For most people, the solution to these issues really isn't an opioid medication for pain control. Additionally, since few people really suffer from a neurotransmitter deficiency, traditional anti-depressants and anti-anxiety drugs will have a limited effect, beyond that of a placebo. This means that learning to be self-supportive and taking self-responsibility for making positive changes are the keys to a pain-free life.

Self-supportive people embody love, feeling supported both internally and externally. Because they feel loved and appreciated, they generate internal feelings of emotional well-being that synchronize their heart and mind, making homeostasis possible.

The differentiation between the two mindsets is eye-opening. It is reported that, by age four, a high proportion of people fall into the self-destructive group, with only a small percentage in the self-supportive cohort. Both nature and nurture influence this divergence. When it comes to treating other people's pain, it can sometimes be challenging, because the self-destructive group wants their doctor, practitioner, or therapist to take on some of their suffering. However, this does nothing to help the patient rewire their threat response, disarm their triggers, or reduce their pain.

The Ripple Effect - Emotional Triggers Turn into Muscle Spasm

Let's look at some of the more common patterns of muscle tension and pain related to common emotional triggers. Below are common examples of emotional triggers manifesting as physical complaints.

- Shoulder pain is often experienced when we feel overburdened by life and our responsibilities, becoming resentful for the added weight. This pain is usually subconscious. Sometimes, it even involves carrying the burdens of other people's pain. This is common in people who are empathic, meaning they are ultra-sensitive, feeling pain that others can't.
- Neck pain plays out when we don't speak our truth or when we have trust issues. Fear and anxiety are frequently stored here.
- Mid back pain accompanies feelings of insecurity, lack of emotional support, and powerlessness.
- Chest wall pain usually accompanies grief.
- Low back pain is associated with guilt, shame, unworthiness, relationship issues, and the fear of not being supported financially.
- Pelvic pain is accompanied by guilt, shame, and rage and is common in people who carry the trauma of sexual abuse and/or struggle with sex addiction.
- Inner thigh pain may reflect a fear of vulnerability. Social anxiety can trigger a threat response in these muscles.

- Outer thigh pain symbolizes frustration and impatience.
- Buttock pain is consistent with Anger, frustration, and rage over dealing with people who are a pain in your butt.

So how does all of this work? According to Dr. Douglas Tataryn of the University of Manitoba, muscles can store emotions, thoughts, and feelings. Once you accept the trigger for the muscle contraction, pain patterns can become wired in. Then, the pain caused by muscle spasms tends to recur or become chronic.

Dr. Tataryn describes four concepts of how we store our unprocessed triggers in the muscles. His paradigm is similar to Dr. Sarno's tension myoneural syndrome (TMS). First, your muscles can save the mind from considerable distress by storing threatening thoughts and feelings. Second, in storing such energy, the muscles become chronically tense, tight, and sore. Third, your awareness of this rigidity in the muscles will soon begin to fade, such that you won't even be aware there is a physical problem. Finally, the release of muscle tension is accompanied by the release of stored emotional energy or thoughts. This can be seen occasionally in treatment when the medical professional taps into a spot associated with stored emotion. When the muscle spasm or tension is released, so is the associated emotion.

This process is called somatoemotional release, which is a therapeutic process that helps the mind and body clear out the residual aspects of past traumas that are associated with negative experiences and negative emotions. If people are not prepared for this, it can be a bit unnerving. With proper coaching, somatoemotional release can be very therapeutic in relieving pain, especially when the underlying trigger is deeply repressed.

Common Causes of Chronic Muscle Spasm

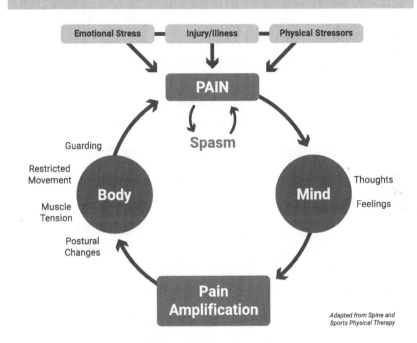

As you can see from the diagram above, there are many reasons we develop chronic muscle spasm leading to the amplification of pain. Some are some physical and some are psychological. Some of the more common reasons include:

- Psychological tension due to negative emotions - such as anger - that stem from our perceptions.
- Trauma ranging from mild to severe in nature. When not consciously addressed, traumatic experiences can lead to a heightened threat response, and possibly even result in PTSD.

- Social conditioning, which is the collection of unspoken social beliefs that we adopt in order to be likable. This can often result in shame, the negative effects of which were explored earlier in the book.
- Environmental stressors, such as poor ergonomics at work, old mattresses and worn-out couches, air and water pollution, toxins, processed food and more.
- Bad habits, such as poor posture and sedentary lifestyle, which prevent us from expelling excess cortisol from our bodies.

Connecting the Dots of Pain and Triggers

In my experience, the final release of the emotional energy is often blocked, because you may be too afraid to release it or you may not remember it. In either scenario, it behooves you to connect the dots between your pain and its triggers by asking yourself this question. When was the last time you felt safe and able to fully relax? Sometimes creating an actual timeline of life events, as well as changes in health status, is helpful in identifying hidden triggers that are very deeply entrenched. People with adverse childhood experiences and significant trauma deal with prolonged stress and dysregulation that can be stored in their bodies for decades. Additionally, their brains are wired to constantly search for clues about where the next threat is coming from. This constant scanning of our environment creates a pattern of hyper-vigilance leading to a heightened threat response, accompanied by all of its physiological ripple effects.

As this process unfolds, you experience the barrage of pain and muscle tension, chronic inflammation, immune dysregulation, and even the possibility of total system shutdown. Until you learn how to effectively deal with your past memories, your pain symptoms will linger, nerves will stay sensitized, and stress hormones (such as cortisol) will remain elevated, all wreaking havoc on your overall state of health.

But this too can change! In fact, there are many paths you can take to improve your ability to self-regulate and reduce pain. If you follow fitness news these days, you may have heard of the Dutch extreme athlete Wim Hof, who encourages his followers to "decondition their mind to recondition their body." This means letting go of old thoughts and beliefs that keep you stuck in the past. When you 'decondition' your mind, you can take the steps to heal and feel more alive. In a sense, when you decondition the mind you engage in the mental pivot or 'counter-thinking.' Resisting the impulse to ignore your thoughts and feelings or judge them as important. They are there for a reason: to help you tune into the messages your body wants you to hear. As part of his radical reconditioning methods, Wim Hof teaches breathing techniques that help to break up entrenched emotional armoring and teach people how to deal with stress. However, please be aware his methods might be a bit 'extreme' for some people to follow. There are some pretty remarkable YouTube videos of Wim Hof in action, if you feel so inclined.

Common sources of everyday stress include:

- Family stressors and relationship changes
- Social stressors
- Changes and transitions
- Chemical stressors (perfumes, new carpets, personal hygiene products, and more)
- Work stressors
- Decision making stressors
- Phobic stressors (irrational fears)
- Physical stressors such as over-exercise and overwork

- Lifestyle stressors
- Environmental stressors
- Pain

You can use this list to start to brainstorm all of the sources of stress that you may be experiencing. There are probably items on your list that you can release. When letting go isn't possible, then reducing the impact of the stressor should be your priority.

Responses to Stress

Every thought, emotion, or environmental trigger yields one of three possible responses:

- Reaction (giving into your emotion)
- Suppression (blocking it out or coping through denial)
- Transformation (awareness allows you to observe the outcome before committing to taking action, thereby allowing you to make something good of a bad situation)

When you know that you are making a clear and deliberate (conscious) decision aligned with your values, then you can go all in with conviction and do your best. This allows you to release all attachment to the emotion. This way, the threat response doesn't get triggered and then become trapped in your mind or body.

As famed psychiatrist, author, and Holocaust survivor Viktor Frankl taught us, you are always able to choose how you feel about any situation. The masters of pain know this. They are the ones who fully experience the rich tapestry of life as it is, without assigning meaning to it. When we allow things to be as they are, there is no judgment or interpretation. This way the threat response can be modulated consciously. The master then turns off their experience or amplifies it at will. They are always present in the moment, eliminating triggering thoughts about past or future events.

Some of us are more emotionally sensitive than others. Emotionally sensitive people react emotionally to most triggers, usually in extreme ways. Common patterns include visceral reactions felt in the body like knots in your stomach, or indigestion, or mental patterns processed in the mind that lead to tension headaches. Some people aren't even aware of why they're consumed by their feelings or why they feel so crappy. But usually these triggers are often prompted by faulty belief systems, usually driven by a core fear. Accepting that we all need to learn to sit with our fears, rather than running from them, will help all of us gain mastery over our pain.

In addition to learning how to deal with our fears, it's also essential that we commit to living a life we love. Be sure not to compromise your happiness for someone else's. Follow your heart, rather than your negative emotions. Trust that your heart will show you the way.

Self-Soothing is Self-Healing

It takes practice to determine what will work best for you to calm your nervous system. Releasing the hold that pain and stress triggers have on you - mental, emotional, physical, or all of the above - requires you to be gentle with yourself. Below are some methods to accomplish this goal.

- Creating a sacred space, where you are surrounded by that things that make you feel safe, is very comforting.
- Scheduling quiet time to do nothing is soothing for your nervous system. Simultaneously listening to relaxing music is helpful as well.

- Singing, chanting mantras and saying affirmations positively influence your subconscious mind.
- Journaling is a beneficial practice, but you need to let your feelings out on paper, without holding back.
- Stretching and foam rolling your muscles are helpful in breaking up tension.
- Epsom salts baths are helpful, because magnesium is a powerful muscle relaxer.
- Exercising with HIIT (high-intensity interval training) techniques helps to discharge excess cortisol. As long as you don't overdo it, HIIT will help you deactivate the threat response.
- Change your exercise routine for each workout.
- Change your environment whenever possible. Walking outside is a wonderful way to change your brain and calm your nervous system.
- Expressing your feelings honestly may not be something you are used to doing, but it may be the most valuable thing you can do. Release your emotions and move on.
- Change your habits, vary your wardrobe, your shoes, and even your route to work every day.
- Lastly, surround yourself with positive people and influences, which is essential because positive energy is contagious.

**"When you can't remember why you hurt,
that's when you're healed."**

- Jane Fonda

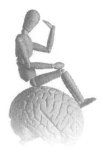

Chapter 6

The Pain Release Process

"The way out of this vicious pain cycle is a wholesale change in how we perceive fear, suffering, and setbacks."

- Rob Heaton

It's a Set-Up

The body's pain mechanisms evolved to report problems; and it works well most of the time. The significant problem with pain is that our minds always demand an explanation. We all want to know why we have pain. More importantly, we want to be reassured that our pain is not a sign of a serious problem. Unfortunately, this isn't always obvious.

Let's consider a young male patient with a herniated disc in his back. He has pain that's consistent with his MRI findings. At the outset, everything appeared straightforward. An epidural steroid injection was performed, as well as the Mckenzie Method of physical therapy but he experienced little to no relief. What gives?

How do we explain why he continues to have pain? This can be a daunting challenge for patients who want definitive explanations for their suffering. However, traditional medical care doesn't always have the answers. When doctors can't produce the expected results, patients often become more anxious, triggering the release of significant quantities of stress hormones. The outcome: their pain intensifies.

We know that pain (especially chronic pain) is not always a reliable indicator of what's going on in the body, because there's always a layer of brain-generated interpretation. The brain critically evaluates every message it receives based on the context in which the pain occurs. Given this, it stands to reason that we feel less pain when we feel calm and safe. On the other hand, if there's a perceived threat looming on the horizon - making us feel stressed, anxious, or fearful - then pain is likely to plague us.

Once the brain gauges the pain signal, and assesses the circumstances, it sends messages that influence nerve sensitivity. Like a knob on an old-fashioned radio receiver, the brain can amplify or decrease pain signals by controlling nerve sensitivity. The brain also sends messages to the organs (via the autonomic nervous system) that control blood flow and the release of various hormones and inflammatory chemicals that greatly impact pain intensity and our healing potential.

As a perception in the brain, pain can be caused by faulty controls and gauges, rather than by actual tissue damage. We need to address these mechanisms, as opposed to solely focusing on the tissue that hurts. With this understanding of pain, we might assume that we can just think away our pain, but it isn't that simple.

Learning how to manage stress and control our thoughts is critical for self-regulation. Our mental and emotional (thinking

114

and feeling) state is the biggest modulator and trigger of physical pain. However, most people have a challenge sorting out their own mental/emotional health.

Additionally, many people have been so stressed out for so long that what they experience is, in effect, a new normal. They don't feel stressed, because the sensations are all that they know. They have no recent memory of living any other way. The reason they have a hard time thinking straight, or being aware of their feelings, is that their system is stuck in fight, flight, or freeze mode, diverting blood and oxygen from the thinking and feeling centers in the brain to other parts of the body.

Indeed, it's a set-up, but most people aren't aware that this is happening. In much the same way that we don't recognize when we have poor posture, people simply can't feel their stress, but they may be able to see it when they look in the mirror. I encourage people to check their faces if they are stressed, distressed, or in moderate to severe pain. Frown lines, squinting in discomfort, tears in the corners of the eyes, and a downturned mouth pursed in an angry scowl are just a few of the unmistakable signs to be aware of.

So, try this. Close your eyes. Open them. Relax. Breathe. Now, visualize an iceberg floating in the ocean. Imagine for a moment that your pain is the uppermost part of the iceberg, buoyed by your hidden feelings and thoughts, which make up the vastly larger chunk hidden under the surface. The iceberg analogy is an apt metaphor for pain, because water symbolizes emotion and the iceberg is a 'chunk' of frozen emotion in the body. When we recognize and release the part that is under the water, which is the foundation, trigger or root cause of the pain, then we can start to dissolve the whole iceberg. 'The Pain Release Process' is like a GPS system helping us locate the underlying target, so we can more effectively navigate it.

The Pain Release Process will help you root out stressful emotional issues that lie hidden under the surface of your pain. The Pain Release Process gets at the core of our 'pain being.' These are the problems we conveniently tuck in our tissues, hoping they won't be brought into the light of day. Pain doesn't have to be caused by easily-diagnosed tissue damage to be real. Physical pain can be driven by psychological triggers, with a psychological root cause as the actual culprit. Don't let any doctor or loved one tell you that your pain is imaginary or 'all in your head.'

Learning how to modulate your brain function is best achieved using a combination of physiological and psychological approaches. Physiological impact can be accomplished through any means of making the painful area feel better or more supported. Massage, bracing, kinesio-taping, the use of ice or heat, and topical salves or essential oils are all helpful. It's also beneficial to practice simple breathing and relaxation exercises to stimulate the parasympathetic nervous system. In fact, anything that gives you hope and confidence that you can get better, will go a long way to helping you calm your nervous system and alleviate your pain.

Learning effective coping strategies is also necessary. On a psychological level, we can learn to positively influence our perception filters (the context of the pain) created by our thoughts, beliefs, feelings, and emotions. By learning to consciously manage our controls and gauges, we can avoid constantly triggering our unconscious autonomic fight-or-flight response. Knowledge and perspective about our beliefs, fears, and behaviors is essential. It's best not to hide in a state of denial, because pain will ultimately find you and target you.

Unfortunately, too few people have been exposed to these insights. As such, people in pain often feel they're at the mercy of what they are told by doctors and healthcare professionals, many of whom operate with outdated ideas and beliefs about what pain is and how to treat it. Additionally, it's important to recognize that everything in life is constantly changing or dying. This is also true of pain; it has the potential to change or even disappear. But, we have to believe this to make it a reality!

Remember, the most powerful predictor for recovery from pain is our expectation that recovery is possible. In discovering how to take control of pain, you must agree to take an active role in reframing the story of your pain, and above all, try to avoid dramatizing it. You can do this by seeking out more comfortable life experiences and positive and inspiring social interactions. This is the most direct route to dampening the circuits of pain and easing the brain's interpretation of what's actually happening in your body.

The Pain Release Process

The Eight Steps to Release Pain

The Pain Release Process (PRP) will be explored in the following pages as part of our pain medicine toolbox. The Pain Release Process (PRP) can help you become more cognizant of the subconscious human drives that pull you out of awareness and self-regulation, keeping you stuck on the proverbial painful 'hamster wheel' of life.

Eight steps to release pain and guide yourself back to health and happiness:

1. Practice self-responsibility.
2. Root out hidden mental and emotional triggers that cause fear.

3. Release three things: past hurts, the need for control, and resistance to change.
4. Reframe your pain story.
5. Rest and reset.
6. Practice self-regulation.
7. Retrain mental habits and physical postures that contribute to pain.
8. Reclaim your power to fully heal.

Step #1 in the Pain Release Process

Practice self-responsibility.

I am fond of the mantra, 'If it's to be, it's up to me.' Pain is not for the faint of heart! What if pain is really a test to see if we're willing to rise above our current circumstances and fulfill our highest potential?

This is where the test gets complicated. I am not referring to acute pain caused by a sudden injury or following a surgical procedure, where pharmaceutical intervention is often warranted. This is different. We are now addressing that part of human nature in which a person falls into victim mode, looking to blame something or someone else for their misery. The answer lies in learning to make mental shifts which require us to recognize that our emotions and thoughts are solely our responsibility. Being accountable for your life and your choices can take various forms, from modifying how you walk, to improving your posture, to manifesting a new job, relationship, or mindset. The secret is that the brain and the body need to change together as a unified whole. This process starts with your decision to make it happen.

When we recognize pain as a wake-up call, we're motivated to make changes. To improve your condition, you don't have to make wholesale changes all at once. You can start with choosing to make small shifts that bring you back to a better state of balance. Learn to listen to what your body is telling you. Then, let those symptoms motivate you to make small changes. Neuroplasticity confirms the brain is capable of constantly changing. This is, in part, why nothing in life is permanent.

Pain is experienced largely based on our perspective. We can agree that we are always able to change our perspective, but taking responsibility for doing so is often challenging. This is the first step in releasing pain. We must take responsibility, and do the hard work, of changing our perspective. This necessary first step is not something we can delegate to our doctors, therapists, or loved ones.

We also need to appreciate that action taken to facilitate change has the same consequences as inaction and avoidance. Health, happiness, and success are all consequences of our choices to take action or shy away. In this light, persistent pain can be viewed as a factor of the consequences of poor lifestyle choices. Releasing pain requires an honest self-appraisal of the various lifestyle factors that contribute to it. Common variables include diet and nutrition, sleep, relaxation, physical activity and exercise, mental stimulation, having a clear sense of purpose, pursuit of creative expression, relationships, and our physical environments.

When you consult a medical professional with pain complaints, recognize that they may neglect to ask about your lifestyle and habits. For many doctors practicing in the traditional American healthcare (insurance) model, they can only consult with patients for ten minutes at a time. Doctors have to cut straight to the point and learn what's bothering you at the moment. With limited time and energy, the doctor needs to identify the crux of your pain, which is paramount to initial diagnosis and treatment.

I would urge you to take self-responsibility, recognize this reality, demand more time from your doctor, and bring up your deeper lifestyle issues as you become aware of them. You also need to be open to embracing changes that are necessary, even though they may throw you out of your comfort zone. Many doctors take the attitude that discussing lifestyle issues, such as diet and physical activity, is a waste of time because most people are simply not willing to change. I hope that you now know why change is crucial to your health and well being and why taking self-responsibility is the first step to living pain free.

The simple truth is that if we recognize what needs adjusting within ourselves, and proactively implement changes to course-correct, we suffer less and experience more joy. This is the essence of self-awareness. It's about being deeply in touch with our own needs, without being afraid to advocate for ourselves.

An example of this is the everyday office worker who sits at a desk most of the day, usually with poor ergonomics. This means that their sitting posture at their desk is sub-optimal, causing them to have to unconsciously adjust their body to fit the desk. Instead, office workers should do their best to make ergonomic changes to their desk set-up to make their time in the office easier on the body.

Sedentary habits are really bad for our health. As a species, we're just not designed to sit all day. As such, sit-stand desks, ergonomic keyboards and chairs are increasingly recommended as a reasonable accommodation for people with back, neck, and arm pain.

Step #2 in the Pain Release Process

Root out hidden mental and emotional triggers that cause fear.

Ralph Waldo Emerson famously said, "Curiosity will conquer fear even more than bravery will." When we explore how to root out our hidden mental and emotional triggers, we're usually referring to internal cognitive distortions (or distorted thinking) and unconscious fears, rather than external environmental threats. Fear can save us from danger, but it can also be illusory, self-generated by the mind, leading to faulty neural pathways in the brain.

'F.E.A.R.' is an acronym for 'False Evidence Appearing Real.' Copy this and write it down. Now put it where you can see it. Read it every time you're scared. Now imagine your strength. Evaluate the real. Be in your truth.

Fear is a construct of the mind that activates when we feel threatened. It triggers us to 'play it small' in life, keeping us confined to our comfort zone. It often becomes an excuse, causing us to avoid seizing what we want to achieve in life. Fear can trigger our innate threat response resulting in anxiety, worry, and obsessive thoughts. Fear stirs us to protect ourselves from further hurt, prompting us to close off and become 'supra-protective,' like a turtle safe in the confines of its shell.

Fear usually arises from uncertainty and our perceived need to control our life circumstances. However, there can be no doubt that, from time to time, life will throw us curve balls, which are growth opportunities and tests of our faith. At the end of the day, our task is to take all of this fear, sit with it, make it our friend, and then transform it into courage.

It's another swing of the pendulum from one extreme to the other. We go from feeling like a victim, looking outward to assign blame for our suffering, to being a champion who owns the power to heal. When we transcend fear, we rise above unconscious thoughts, beliefs, and reactions that previously limited us to a fear-based and often painful reality.

When we accomplish this, we begin to feel truly safe in the world and in our own skin. We can embody the spirit of courage, which gives us enhanced physical and mental resources to experience the world differently. With these new insights, developed by integration of the mind and the body, we can defeat the mental patterns that previously led us down a path of pain and self-defeat. Instead, we can aspire to achieve optimal health and self-empowerment.

Step #3 in the Pain Release Process

Release three things: past hurts, the need for control, and resistance to change.

"Accept your past without regret, handle your present with confidence, and face your future without fear."

- Unknown

'Letting go' can easily trigger the fear response. When we release something or someone from our lives, leaving it or them behind, we can become intensely afraid of what might be substituted. This is fear of the unknown. This is a fairly common pattern I see in patients who experience pain flare-ups when they are faced with letting go of a habit.

This reminds me of a young professional in her mid-thirties, who had recently moved to the area for a new job. Her previous physician had treated her non-traumatic back and neck pain for several years with opioid medication. She came to me expecting I would continue this same course of treatment.

It was clear at the first visit that she had become accustomed to taking multiple doses of opioid pain medication each day. I reassured her that her medical records reflected a normal MRI of the back and neck. I explained to her that I rarely prescribe opioids for benign chronic pain, nor do I recommend it. Further, I advised her that there was no clear tissue pathology to warrant the use of opioid pain medications. Finally, I explained that I do not recommend treating pain as a symptom.

She was skeptical, but agreed to a course of physical therapy, with the goal of identifying ergonomic factors that might be contributing to her pain. She returned one month later in follow up. I again suggested to her that opioids were not an ongoing treatment option, because her condition simply didn't warrant it. I spent a considerable amount of time explaining to her why this type of drug is not a healthy option for many patients with chronic pain. As I explained all of this,I could see her face getting red and her emotions becoming edgy. Right before my eyes, she went into a state of panic, becoming very defensive, saying 'If you're going to take away my medication, then what are you going to give me instead?'

The tricky thing about fear is that it makes us cling to what we know, even if it keeps us stuck in a rut, no matter how bad it makes us feel. We tend to embrace complacency, that familiar ogre that lurks within all of us. Of course, some people are more ready to exercise the courage to overcome it.

Getting unstuck requires us to remember our injury or trauma and reconsider whether we have to hold on to the story that we attach to our suffering. We don't need to get over the past, we just need to get past it. This does not come naturally or easily to many people in our topsy-turvy world. Letting go and moving on requires us to think and do things differently.

Visualize fear of change as a powerful magnet designed to hold you in place, keeping you just as you are. Releasing the hold that fear has on us is unsettling, bringing us face-to-face with the strongest emotional drivers of human nature: love, fear, and rage.

In the pages to come, you will explore a number of recommendations for letting go and embracing change.

First, 'embrace curiosity' about what is possible. This gives us hope that a better solution to our pain problem can be found. We may develop a fresh new perspective or try a new treatment approach. This can help reduces stress, so we can think more clearly.

Second, 'squash negativity' by questioning invisible, irrational, and unproductive thoughts. These are the 'ANTS' mentioned earlier. Author Byron Katie teaches a method of self-inquiry, which urges us to investigate the following questions. "Is this thought true? Can I be absolutely sure it's true? How do I react when I think this way? And lastly, who would I be without this thought?" As we ask these questions, we tend to react less to the stress created by these old thought patterns.

Third, 'shrink the mountain to a molehill.' Many people catastrophize their pain. While it's understandable, this emotional reaction steeps our brain in chronic pain and causes it to employ mechanisms, such as central sensitization and sympathetic overdrive, that magnify our suffering. By changing our perspective and consciously overriding these automatic responses, we can remove the 'magnifying glass' we previously focused on our pain, making our issues much easier to overcome.

Fourth, 'swim in the deep end,' by acknowledging your hidden emotions. This means sitting with them until they no longer maintain their hold over you. This is crucial, as these feelings take up valuable space in our heads, zapping our energy, and keeping us stuck in the past. Holding onto these hidden emotions keeps us 'locked up', which manifests physically in the body as chronic muscle tension or 'tension myoneural syndrome' (TMS).

Fifth, 'anchor into the future' by creating realistic goals and a clear positive vision of the future, which can help you let go of pain from the past. Remember that the brain has difficulty engaging in conflicting beliefs. If you're focused on a better tomorrow, you will be less likely to remain stuck in yesterday. This is certainly challenging, but when it comes to envisioning your future, think of the maxim, 'Fake it til you make it.' Feeling the future in your cells is the key to manifesting a better life.

Sixth, 'discard remnants of the past' by simplifying and lightening your load. Discard unnecessary baggage and try to carry fewer burdens. This helps you to move forward. A neat ritual for releasing your past hurts is the act of designating a 'Satan's suitcase,' such as an old suitcase or box, where you store the artifacts from your painful past. Then you put this suitcase to the side, until you're ready to let it go completely. Think of it as putting your past pain behind you, because it's trapped away, you'll no longer be able to see or feel it.

Seventh, 'repair relationships and practice forgiveness.' Many interpersonal connections become 'frayed' and mired in conflict due to past hurts. When we make amends for our part in a relationship gone badly, it's very liberating, releasing the pain from the past. When this is not possible or appropriate, then forgiveness becomes our most powerful healing tool. Forgiveness is a funny thing. The things we hold on to clearly weigh us down and keep us stuck in threat mode, perpetuating stress, and pain. Genuine and heartfelt forgiveness can move us to believe that we have more to gain by forgiving, than from staying angry. The paradox of forgiveness is that we think we are forgiving the other person, but we are really forgiving ourselves for our role in the painful situation. Self-forgiveness is freeing. It's important from any perspective.

We live in a world in which our senses are constantly bombarded with unrealistic images of how we should look and behave. The aspect of self-imposed pressure to conform to these external and internal messages can be overwhelming and even become a kind of self-injury. Feeling that we 'don't measure up,' 'aren't good enough,' or 'will never amount to anything,' can cause shame and lead us to self-sabotage. In these instances, self-forgiveness is the greatest gift we can give ourselves. It's an act of self-love and self-preservation.

Eighth, 'pass on the perfect.' Perfectionism and the need to control circumstances in our lives (and the lives of others) are common emotional triggers of pain. The perfectionist pushes themselves to the brink and the 'control freak' pushes others. These are both traits that drive people to attain success at all costs. Yet, they always come at a price. As we now know, they make us susceptible to pain.

Ninth, 'give up your grief.' Letting go of grief is a challenge for many people. In my practice, I have seen firsthand the power that unresolved grief has as a pain generator. Like fear, anger, and rage, grief is a challenging negative emotion that masquerades as pain.

For many years, I treated a lovely woman in her eighties. After the death of her husband of 60 years, she developed a severe case of shingles on her chest. Because of the stress of her loss, and the intense reactions of grief, her immune system became suppressed, leading to development of a form of chronic pain called post-herpetic neuralgia. We attempted to make her comfortable using all of the available topical and oral medications, but her grief was so intense and persistent that her pain became hard to manage. At my insistence, she finally agreed to go to grief counseling. With that, her coping strategies improved, her pain lessened, and her overall health improved. Grief is such a powerful emotion that we often hear about couples in which one partner dies shortly after the other, because the pain of the broken heart is too hard to bear.

Step #4 in the Pain Release Process

Reframe your pain story.

Most of us who experience pain allow our condition to dictate our mental attitude. Our pain triggers emotions of frustration, worry, fear, and anger. As such, we become anxious for our condition to improve. However, since all pain and distress starts at the cellular level, it is important for us to focus on good feelings and thoughts. This allows for optimal cellular communication, allowing your body's wisdom to take the helm. It is crucial to reframe your frustration with pain and focus instead on healing.

In his children's book about self-mastery, *Zach Gets Frustrated*, William Mulcahy teaches kids how to learn healthy ways of dealing with frustration. Mr. Mulcahy's paradigm of 'Name it, Tame it, and Reframe It' makes for a wonderful tool for dealing with pain. Allow me to demonstrate how this process works.

'Naming your pain' helps you to become more aware of its underlying causes. It's also a playful exercise that stimulates your right brain function, giving you access to more creative solutions to problems. This way you don't get mired in analysis paralysis.

One way to name your pain in a way that can remove the trigger is to use humor. Consider giving silly names to your triggers. When we name our pain in this way, making it seem more benign, it can draw away some of its power over us. Remember that we don't want to feed negative images and perceptions to our subconscious mind. When people come to see me with pain issues, they often have trouble finding the words to describe their pain. When we don't have a consistent language for pain, we have a hard time relating to it. As we develop new understandings of pain as a messenger of the mind-body connection, we will need to work on new ways of creating a language for it.

'Taming your pain' takes you out of your automatic fear-based response patterns. Developing a more relaxed attitude brings you into the present moment, allowing you to sit with it, empowering you to more authentically connect with the messages your body is sending you. Utilize simple breathing techniques and other soothing, self-care strategies, such as progressive body relaxation (The Body Scan Meditation), Epsom salt baths, essential oils, spending time in nature, prayer, and listening to music. The Body Scan Meditation will be presented in more detail in Chapter 8 - Health as a Habit. These practices will help get you out of your head and back into your body, where you need to be if you wish to reverse the effects of stress, frustration, pain, and other negative states.

'Reframing your pain' becomes possible once you recognize that you can eliminate the fear and frustration associated with it. Then, and only then, can you change your perspective. Human beings are susceptible to 'framing effects,' meaning that we respond to situations based on how they're presented to us. You can now 're-contextualize' your pain using everything you've learned about the brain and nervous system, thereby allowing you to move into a place of true healing.

We've established that nothing in life is permanent, that we can choose our thoughts, and that we can take action to change anything in our life that's not working for us. Simple examples of reframing include: 'This too shall pass' and 'Everything has a way of working itself out.'

Reframing through positive affirmations is a wonderful way to bypass the subconscious mind and our automatic reactive nature. This can help cut off the roots of our suffering. Reframing or rewriting our pain story doesn't change the facts of the narrative. It allows us to see the facts from a different, more enlightened, and more empowered perspective. We can begin to see ourselves and others in a different light, helping us to reduce the shame and blame that often make up the plot of our pain narrative. We can then take ownership of the story, telling it from a more balanced and compassionate point of view. This retelling transforms us from the role of a victim to the hero of our own story.

Step #5 in the Pain Release Process

Rest and reset.

**"Jason Bourne concentrated on rest and mobility.
From somewhere in his forgotten past, he understood that
recovery depended upon both and he applied rigid
discipline to both."**

- Robert Ludlum, The Bourne Identity

Does art imitate life or does life imitate art? We can learn a lot from the stories depicted in movies, because they are universal tales of human suffering and our remarkable ability to overcome obstacles. In many of these stories, a secret government agent accomplishes his or her 'impossible' mission, then has to go 'dark,' while the blowback occurs, and the story unfolds. In the same way, we need to develop patterns of taking action, while balancing with adequate rest. This is challenging for many who attempt to proceed through life relentlessly, without allowing for sufficient recovery time.

When it comes to healing an acute injury, or resolving an overuse syndrome, science demonstrates that 'relative rest' as opposed to strict bed rest is an essential ingredient in any healing recipe. It allows us to reset the nervous system's response to injury, pain, and stress and reduces direct tissue damage caused by overload. People often mistakenly believe that rehabilitation is only about physical exercise. However, the injured body part needs to feel supported in order to heal. 'Relative rest' allows us to give injured tissues a break, while we continue to exercise our healthy, uninjured body parts.

Some people have faulty notions about the negative effects of rest. They believe that, if they rest, they will become overweight and out of shape. Remember that caloric intake is far more relevant to our weight than exercise. Thus, when we have to rest in order to heal, we can choose to reduce our caloric intake. Looking at sleep and nutrition are also important considerations in the early healing phase of an injury. Without these supportive measures, pain can become chronic. Diets with the proper balance of protein, vegetables and healthy fats are essential. Core nutrients such as vitamin C, vitamin A, vitamin D, zinc, and magnesium also promote healing. We will discuss this more in the Chapter 8, called 'Health as a Habit.'

Another incorrect assumption about rest is that we need strict bed rest in order to heal. This myth has been debunked. It's generally accepted now that 'early mobilization' has replaced strict bed rest. This principle applies to everything from back pain to tendon ruptures to fracture healing. Considerable scientific evidence shows that in the early stages of healing the stimulation of gentle movement is a crucial part of triggering and maintaining a healing response. This also helps to prevent the painful loop of fear avoidance, which we see so often in chronic pain patients. For these people, it hurts to move so they decide that the only way to control their pain is to avoid moving. This can also occur when they're so anxious about their pain getting worse, that they walk around in a braced or guarded posture. It's as if they are waiting for the other shoe to drop!

We need to strike a balance between rest and mobilization, so that we can stay active, without putting too much stress on our injured tissues. Injuries to our feet, knees, and hips are difficult to heal because it's harder to rest these areas.

It's also challenging to recognize when our injuries have fully healed, because we have stopped exercising. Returning to exercise after injury needs to be done in a graded fashion, so we don't re-aggravate the injured tissue. Timing of return to exercise is complicated and everyone is unique. Consulting your physician, physical therapist, or certified personal trainer will be critical in developing the best plan for you to return to activity.

In my experience, cross-training with water exercise programs or swimming can be very helpful in recovering from lower extremity injuries, because it eliminates gravity, allowing for graded muscle activation in a supported environment. It also completely changes the context of exercise and pain, because we don't usually associate the pool as a place where we might get injured. Caution needs to be taken to gradually increase time in the pool, because of the added resistance of the water.

Upper extremity injuries from golf and tennis are also challenging to recover from, because of overuse, poor form, and the fact that we return too quickly to the course or court. This makes healing of torn tendons and irritated tissue incomplete and makes us more susceptible to re-injury.

Healing these kinds of injuries requires several things:

1. Decrease tissue load by reducing frequency of stress and improving form or modifying the equipment.
2. Reduce inflammation in general by managing the stress response effectively (this is part of the reset process).
3. Consider regenerative medicine techniques, such as platelet-rich plasma (PRP), in lieu of steroid injections.

As we will soon learn steroid injections can be helpful for painful arthritis and inflamed joints. However, use them with caution in tendons and soft tissues, because ultimately, they lead to tissue breakdown, which further enhances risk of re-injury.

On an emotional level, coming to grips with the need to 'relatively rest' and reset is also challenging. Many of us enjoy exercise, using it as a way to manage stress and maintain our mood. We often have the attitude that if a little activity is good, then more is better. Beware! There is a delicate balance between effort and rest, which requires us to pay close attention to early warning signs, such as mild discomfort and swelling. This is especially true with relatively minor symptoms like plantar fasciitis, IT band syndrome, shin splints, tennis elbow, and rotator cuff tendonitis. We usually don't expect these minor issues to require us to rest and reset, but they usually do.

Step #6 in the Pain Release Process

Practice self-regulation.

"Between stimulus and response, there is a space. In that space is our power to choose our response. In our response lies our growth and freedom."

- Viktor Frankl

Self-regulation is defined as our ability to behave in ways that support our health and long-term survival, but are also in keeping with our highest values. Understanding all aspects of this is important because violation of our values invariably causes bad feelings, which work counter to self-regulation. On an emotional level, self-regulation allows us to calm down when we are upset and uplift ourselves when we are suffering. On a physiological level, our feelings and emotions move us by sending chemical messages and electrical signals to our muscles, preparing us for action. According to relationship expert Dr. Steven Stosny, our emotions motivate us to do one of three things in any situation: approach, avoid, or attack.

- 'Approach emotions' promote interest and a sense of fun, as well as compassion and trust. These are essential for loving relationships. Approach emotions also lead to behaviors such as openness to learning new things, socializing, cooperating, and setting appropriate limits. Approach emotions release feel good hormones such as oxytocin, which help us relax, bond, and reduce stress, thereby reducing pain.
- 'Avoid emotions' cause distancing and social isolation. They perpetuate resistance to change, making it harder to

seek help. Avoid emotions are at the root of many self-defeating behaviors. They often create muscle tension and guarding, which can become painful habit patterns.

- 'Attack emotions' often undermine and harm us by stirring up anger and rage throwing us into reactive modes of fight or flight which trigger pain. These negative emotions promote self-defeating behaviors such as manipulation, threatening, and bullying, and can lead to autoimmune conditions in the body.

Dr. Stosny goes on to say, "we give psychological meaning to anything that makes us feel uncomfortable. Self-regulation is easier when we focus our energy on our values, rather than our feelings, because feelings are fickle. When we focus on feelings, they often get amplified and distorted, triggering our fear response. Focusing on our values keeps us feeling better about ourselves and focused on the positive solutions. Self-regulation also calls us to appreciate delayed gratification, be aware of our own emotional state, express our needs and feelings, and calm ourselves and others appropriately."

Step #7 in the Pain Release Process

Retrain mental habits and physical postures that contribute to pain.

"Change your thoughts and change your world."

- Norman Vincent Peale

Our bodies physically react and change in response to every thought that we have. This is a result of our chemical messengers-neurotransmitters, which facilitate communication between our muscles, nervous system, organs, and cells. The power of thought has been proven in studies. There's growing evidence that we can improve almost anything, from our vision to our fitness, by intentionally directing our thoughts. However, because this phenomenon is totally free, the pharmaceutical companies don't want you to know about it, as people might start eschewing their expensive, frequently ineffective, and sometimes harmful products.

Thoughts can even program our cells through proteins called peptides, which are molecules that are linked with specific thoughts and emotions. When these peptides surge through our body and connect with specific receptors on our cells, our cells adapt. If we bombard our cells with negative peptides, then we bias the system this way, making it harder to receive positive peptides. This programs the cells to keep us stuck in negativity. Since our cells naturally regenerate every two months, we can actually retrain the system by using strategies such as gratitude, mindfulness practices, and positive thinking.

As spiritual guru Deepak Chopra says, "our cells are always eavesdropping on our mind." This means we can affect how our genes are expressed through our thought patterns. The science of epigenetics further demonstrates that our genes can be switched on or off, based on our life experiences and how we perceive them.

Our thoughts and perceptions control our biology. Through a combination of our thoughts and lifestyle choices, we get to choose the inputs we provide. Making this process conscious, rather than habitual, is the key to personal power and ultimate health.

The Buddhist practice of RAIN, which you explored in Chapter 4, is useful in teaching us to leave our mind out of our perception of pain. In these exercises, when pain arises in our body, we investigate whether it comes with a sensation or an emotion or a thought. Then, we let it pass without getting attached or identifying with it. Like a cloud floating across the sky, it slowly drifts away. This is how we can start to exercise restraint over the mind. Focusing awareness on the pain at the level of physical sensation keeps the pain in our body and out of our mind. There, we can meet our pain 'head on.'

Step #8 in the Pain Release Process

Reclaim your power to fully heal.

"We reclaim our power by loving the parts of ourselves we were once taught to hate."

- Bryant H. McGill

Pain is not our enemy. Learning to love every part of us, even the parts that hurt, is a requirement for healing. Taking self-responsibility for identifying the messages embedded in your pain, as well as growing your awareness of your automatic triggers, will free you from suffering.

These two actions force us to grow and evolve, and teach us to effectively cope with the challenging and unpleasant aspects of life. In mastering both our emotional and physical natures, we can unite the mind and body. This brings our innate special powers of an open mind and open heart to the healing table. Integrating these two special forces allows us to learn to love all parts of us - the broken and the whole - and reclaim our power to fully heal!

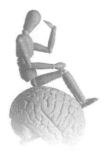

Chapter 7

The Pain Treatment Toolbox - 'When to Treat and What to Treat'

"I am still learning."

- Michelangelo

Treat the Problem, Not the Symptom

Pain is a part of life, but treating pain is not a one-size-fits-all approach. Everyone's pain is different. New approaches are being developed to treat pain, trauma, and inflammation. As the opioid crisis takes on epidemic proportions and healthcare costs continue to explode, the traditional concepts of pain management are fading. The paradigm that I advance in this book, along with the efforts of thousands of like-minded practitioners, are the vanguard of a revolution.

I will be the first to admit that doctors, myself included, don't have all of the answers for why you hurt and suffer. The new paradigm of treating pain, of which I am a leading proponent, demands that we ask the right questions and listen for the right answers, so that we can identify the appropriate tool for each problem. Ultimately, we need a solutions-oriented paradigm, rather than the treatment approach focused on problems (symptoms) that is still common today.

Treating pain as a symptom, without 'looking under the hood' for clear explanations, is what has led to the healthcare crisis we face today. A new model of pain assessment and treatment - in which doctors and patients work collaboratively to search for clues to hidden physical, emotional, and lifestyle triggers - is the way of the future. New tools are needed to help patients and doctors navigate the complexities of the mind-body connection. This is what I call 'pain literacy.'

Medication Management

Currently, medication management is the most common form of treatment for both acute and chronic pain. Over-the-counter medications include analgesics such as Aspirin, acetaminophen (Tylenol), as well as nonsteroidal anti-inflammatory drugs (NSAIDS) such as ibuprofen (Advil/Motrin) and naproxen (Aleve). Medications that are used today to reduce pain temporarily, but which require prescriptions, include opioids with some form of codeine, muscle relaxers, short-term oral steroids, low-dose naltrexone, antidepressants, and 'anti-seizure' drugs, including Gabapentin, Topamax, and Lyrica. There are stronger opioids as well, such as Morphine, Fentanyl, Dilaudid, and others.

Of course, tens of millions of people rely on one or more of these types of drugs to get through their day. However, medication has become a crutch for so many, even in the cases of the non-habit-forming drugs. The reality is that no drug, either prescription or over-the-counter, can solve pain problems on a long-term basis. Moreover, they are potentially 'habit forming.' Beside the potential for addiction and overdose, opioids present other special considerations. Such phenomena include drug tolerance (decreased effectiveness over time), opioid hyperalgesia (paradoxical increase in pain), constipation, as well as immune and hormonal (estrogen and testosterone) suppression, which is seen equally in both men and women.

As a physician, I am not 'anti-medication.' However, when these medications are used to treat chronic pain, they only provide limited relief, and only for so long as you take them. Over the three decades of treating people in pain, I've learned that medication is best used as a short-term bridge to buy time to search for the best solutions and help you to get moving and engaged in life again. Imagine walking around on crutches after a torn ACL, but never doing any physical therapy to heal the injury. This is exactly the trap that gets so many well-intentioned people, who are genuinely suffering, but don't know there is a better way than long-term medication usage to overcome their pain.

We're at a critical time of change in healthcare. Everything's up for grabs, and new ideas about how to manage health, and not disease, are coming to the forefront. More holistic ways of addressing pain, and its true root causes, are becoming more widely accepted and people are increasingly taking to heart the benefits of living healthier lifestyles. In order to outsmart the 'medication management cycle,' there are many medical treatment options that I will help you to explore.

Interventional Pain Therapies

As a physiatrist, I am uniquely qualified to treat the whole person. Throughout much of the book, I have guided you through an exploration of mind-body medicine, including the emotional causes of pain, pain habits, health habits, and more. I am aware that some people may find some of my ideas about pain to be a bit unconventional, even somewhat 'woo-woo.' However, it is important to remember that there is plenty of science to support my overarching concepts.

With that said, it my sincere belief that traditional pain therapies have a role to play. When used in conjunction with the ideas I have introduced in the book, we can help people achieve healing that has previously eluded them under the traditional healthcare model. In the same way that gunshot wounds (to name an extreme example) cannot be healed by our thoughts and habits alone, many conditions presenting with pain as a primary symptom do require more hands-on medical treatments.

Many physiatrists today are trained in interventional pain therapies that are designed to provide fast relief for people suffering from painful conditions. We can perform a variety of procedures, including injections to quickly relieve pain, such as nerve blocks and epidural steroid injections that alleviate pain from herniated discs and nerve compression. We also perform a variety of joint injections including facet joint injections as well as sacroiliac joint injections for spinal pain caused by arthritis of the spinal and pelvic joints. Radiofrequency ablation (RFA) is another minimally invasive procedure that provides more lasting relief for chronic arthritis of the neck and low back. In severe cases of nerve pain, we can even implant spinal cord stimulators, which act to pace impulses along the spinal cord, blocking pain from traveling to the brain. Some physiatrists are also skilled in the use of musculoskeletal ultrasound for both diagnosis and the treatment of tendon, muscle, and joint-related issues. These are all tools that I use every day in my practice to relieve pain and restore function.

And Now a Word About Inflammation

One commonality of many pain syndromes is inflammation. Understanding inflammation is important because it's the root cause of all degenerative and chronic diseases, including heart disease and cancer. As you've learned in the book, inflammation can help us by triggering a healing response, but it can also hurt us. Learning about this will help you make better lifestyle choices. There are two distinct types of inflammation: acute and chronic. This should sound familiar, because it has the same nature as pain.

Typically, acute inflammation is a local condition caused by injury or wear and tear in a particular tissue. Chronic inflammation, on the other hand, is a systemic condition that can trigger a wide range of harmful downstream and upstream effects. It's like a tidal wave in the body moving in two directions at once. Chronic inflammation is the very same process caused by the chronic stress and threat response. They are flip sides of the same coin.

Systemic effects of inflammation and stress trigger genes to activate, predisposing you to a long slate of degenerative conditions, including diabetes, obesity, cancer, heart and vascular disease, Alzheimer's, stomach and intestinal issues, asthma, thyroid disease, skin conditions, and fertility issues.

Inflammation takes a toll on our organs, weakening our heart muscle, raising our blood sugars, affecting our mitochondria's ability to produce energy, and reducing the absorption of nutrients, causing premature osteoporosis, neuropathy, and other problems.

Regenerative Medicine vs. Corticosteroid Injections

Regenerative Medicine is a relatively new field in the pain treatment realm. It is still not considered mainstream by most health insurance companies, as well as Medicare. However, the esteemed Mayo Clinic identifies regenerative medicine "as a game changing area of medicine with the potential to fully heal damaged tissues and organs, offering hope to people who have conditions that are today considered beyond repair." The concepts of regenerative medicine are not new, but the clinical applications are improving with the use of image guidance (x-ray and ultrasound) and the development of unique ways of activating the cells and directing them to the damaged tissue.

The mainstay of regenerative medicine today is PRP, which stands for 'platelet-rich plasma.' PRP (not to be mistaken for the Pain Release Process) is comprised of platelets and signaling proteins (called growth factors) that come from your own blood. Like a symphony conductor, these signalling proteins direct our cells to heal injured or degenerated tissues. When people come in for PRP injections, my staff draws blood from their arm and places it in a special centrifuge to spin out the red and most of the white cells, leaving the platelets and the platelet-related growth factors. Platelets are best known for their role in blood clotting. For example, when you accidentally cut yourself, the hundreds of proteins (growth factors) in platelets are critical in clot formation as well as in the body's healing mechanisms. Platelets serve many functions including binding and releasing bacteria and viruses, which reduces the risk of infection. They also play a role in modulating inflammation. The magic of PRP therapy is in how it works with our body's natural repair mechanisms. It has been shown to improve cell proliferation and collagen production, facilitate DNA/gene expression, and facilitate the formation of new healthy tissue by establishing a supportive tissue matrix in injured tendons and joints.

Before the development of PRP, physicians (myself included) used cortisone injections to relieve moderate to severe muscle, tendon, bursa, and joint-related pain due to inflammation. Unlike cortisone injections, PRP works differently because it not only reduces inflammation, but it also promotes tissue healing and regeneration by delivering hundreds of valuable bioactive signaling proteins to the injured area of the body. This, in turn, catalyzes your innate healing response.

Both cortisone injections and PRP injections can provide pain relief. However, cortisone injections have a 'dark' side. I am not referring to the use of performance-enhancing anabolic steroids that athletes use to convert proteins into lean muscle mass. This is different. The steroids we typically inject into inflamed tissue are corticosteroids, which work by disrupting a specific step in the inflammatory cascade. They are targeted to specific tissue(s), and they can also work systemically when needed. Corticosteroid injection are advantageous because they work quickly, and their effects can last for a long time. However, corticosteroid injections also break down your tissues, weaken and tear tendons, and contribute to the degeneration of joints, especially if they're injected repeatedly. Moreover, they can cause fat atrophy in the skin at the injection site, and potentially break down bone. While corticosteroid injections are generally safe and effective, they are often quick fixes that can mask pain, rather than repairing injured tissue.

PRP on the other hand, stimulates cellular growth and tissue regeneration slowly, re-building the injured or degenerated area over time. In general, we expect people to be sore for about three to four days post-injection. We typically expect to see an early response to PRP injections after about three weeks.

PRP injections are dramatically less risky than cortisone injections, but the cost is higher, since insurance currently doesn't cover it. PRP injections are now commonly performed using ultrasound or X-ray guidance into any joint, ligament, or tendon ranging from the bottom of your feet to the neck and shoulders. While it less commonly done, PRP injections can also be performed for painful lumbar discs.

There are a growing number of studies that show significantly favorable results of PRP in alleviating pain over the long-term for conditions such as osteoarthritis of the knee and shoulder, tendonitis of the elbow, rotator cuff tears, plantar fasciitis, and Achilles tendon tears. It's important to know that, before undergoing regenerative medicine therapies, such as PRP, it is recommended to stop NSAIDS, aspirin, and fish oil about seven to ten days prior to the procedure. All of these substances can affect your platelets and you don't want to take a chance that they will alter the effects of the treatment in any way. There are also special considerations for the use of PRP for patients on blood thinners and people with low platelet counts. These special conditions would need to be addressed with your treating physician.

Other Important Players in the Regenerative Medicine Lineup

There are a growing number of regenerative medicine options. For example, 'amniotic membrane therapy' is an injection using freeze-dried amniotic membrane from the placenta. This injection is similar to PRP, since the solution delivers growth factors and signalling proteins to the target site. This modality is typically much more costly than PRP and the volume of the injection is much smaller. We consider this an alternative to PRP when the patients either can't come off of their blood thinners or they have a low platelet count in their blood. Another treatment option is 'combination therapy,' which involves incorporating PRP and amniotic membrane therapy. However, be aware that there are no specific studies to date showing that combination therapy is more effective than either technique on its own.

Viscosupplementation injections are not considered 'regenerative,' but Euflexxa can be combined with PRP to provide an added temporary benefit. Viscosupplementation injections are currently approved by some insurance companies for the treatment of moderate osteoarthritis of the knee. I liken these injections to an 'oil change for your knee.' The knee has hydraulic features and this injection works to make the joint fluid thicker, providing you with more 'cushion' inside your knee. When we combine viscosupplementation with PRP, insurance will not cover it, but the additional cost is relatively low. Patients with severe cases of degenerative osteoarthritis might benefit the most from this combination therapy.

Regenerative injections can also include fat grafting and stem cells derived from bone marrow. These therapies are more invasive, requiring the harvesting of fat through a mini-liposuction procedure. Alternatively, we can tap the reservoir of stem cells in the bone marrow of your sacrum to obtain the bone marrow concentrate. When you have a really stubborn condition, these more advanced techniques could be considered.

In most facilities, regenerative procedures are done the same day in your doctor's office and then you can go home immediately afterwards to rest. It is recommended you take it easy for three to four days post treatment and then gradually resume activity. Ice applied to the injection site is helpful to reduce pain and swelling.

'Prolotherapy' injections were the early forerunner in the regenerative medicine lineup. Prolotherapy was innovated by Dr. Hemwall and Dr. Hackett in the 1950s. I had the great fortune to learn from Dr. Hemwall, when he was still practicing at age ninety. Prolotherapy is an amazingly powerful, but simple, treatment for injured, torn, and lax ligaments. We also use prolotherapy to treat hypermobile joints. Prolotherapy is comprised of a mixture of highly concentrated sugar water (dextrose) and lidocaine (numbing medication), which is then injected into targeted tendons, ligaments, and joints. Prolotherapy is designed to tighten elastic tissues, promoting joint support and stability. I have been using prolotherapy on a daily basis since 1992 to treat a variety of painful conditions. The patients who benefit the most are hypermobile. These people either were born with ligament laxity or they developed lax ligaments from injury or overuse.

As I discussed in the introduction, prolotherapy helped me to recover from my serious neck injury. Along with surgery and a lot of self-care, it helped me get my life back. I usually perform these injections under ultrasound or X-ray guidance. People who benefit the most from prolotherapy include those who are recovering from trauma (as in my case) and athletes with stubborn ligament strains. People with hypermobility syndromes such as Ehlers-Danlos (EDS) should also consider prolotherapy as a treatment option. EDS is typically an inherited collagen disorder that results in ligaments being too lax, meaning they lack the necessary support for the joints, leading to chronic pain issues.

Other Important Pain Therapies

Physical therapy is a critical part of any pain program. However, if used incorrectly, it could make the pain worse. The field of physical therapy is going through a lot of changes and not all physical therapists are appropriate for each individual's condition. It's important to select the right therapist for the right problem. You definitely want to see a physical therapist skilled in the best techniques to address your needs.

For example, people who limp or have poor posture, faulty movement patterns, and weak muscles, ideally need a physical therapist trained in neuromuscular re-education. These techniques address the altered wiring that causes some muscles to stay weak, painful, and tight after an injury heals. Neuromuscular re-education also helps correct the problematic compensation patterns that develop when one hurts. Appropriate muscle re-education includes-normalizing muscle firing patterns, core strengthening, gait training, and breathing exercises to strengthen the diaphragm. It is very important that therapy services be provided within the context of a supportive therapeutic relationship, because feeling safe is essential to healing any pain problem and shortening therapy time.

There is a growing understanding of how and why our core body of muscles is essential to living without pain, because it links our breath with our posture. Having a strong core doesn't mean that you need 'six-pack' stomach muscles. Rather, it means that you can generate increased abdominal pressure to protect your back from compression and bending injuries that lead to herniated discs. Physical therapists trained in a European technique called Dynamic Neuromuscular Stabilization (DNS) and Postural Restoration (PRI) are particularly tuned in to how the core works relative to your breath and posture.

Additionally, there is growing awareness of the importance of breath control in activating the parasympathetic nervous system - through the action of the vagus nerve - to shut down the threat response and prevent the cascade of psycho-neuro-hormonal changes that accompany stress and fear. You now have some new skills to help you improve your breathing and your core. Any time spent on improving your breathing patterns and establishing conscious breath control will reduce your pain, lower stress, and improve your health.

If you have a herniated disc, then you ideally want to consult McKenzie-trained physical therapists, who are certified to assess and treat herniated discs in the back and neck. The McKenzie therapy approach centers around the notion of 'centralization of pain.' If you have sciatica, with pain shooting down your leg, or if you have a pinched nerve in your neck that shoots pain down your arm, then this therapy mainly uses repetitive extension movements designed to move the pain out of the painful limb and into the center of the spine. McKenzie therapy works wells in reducing the size of herniated discs and facilitating recovery without surgery. In my experience, it works best in combination with epidural corticosteroid injections. There is a synergistic effect between the McKenzie therapy and the epidural injections, as one works on the structural component of the herniated disc, while the other focuses on the chemically mediated inflammation.

Trigger point dry needling is another physical therapy modality that is helpful in treating chronic myofascial pain syndromes. It is similar to trigger point injections performed by physicians and involves inserting acupuncture-type needles in critical points in the body. This helps to breakup painful areas of muscle tension and spasm. Trigger point dry needling is most effective in chronic muscular disorders. It is painful but effective. However, not all physical therapists are qualified to perform these techniques. If you have chronic myofascial issues, you would want to seek out a therapist specifically trained in this modality.

Visceral manipulation is a manual technique developed by Jean Pierre Barral of the Barral Institute. One of the ideas behind this technique is that internal scar tissue from abdominal and pelvic procedures can affect how our organs move, impacting our posture and movement patterns. Unfortunately, the impact that scar tissue has on pain is underappreciated. Both internal and external scars can cause pain and postural alterations. If you have had extensive abdominal or pelvic surgery, and have persistent pain, consider seeing a physical therapist who specializes in visceral manipulation.

Visceral manipulation also helps with the internal scars, while 'neuroprolotherapy,' or scar injections, help with external scar tissue. This is a technique developed 'down under' in New Zealand by Dr. John Lyftgot. It involves injecting a very diluted solution of Mannitol and Lidocaine into and around scars to release small trapped nerve fibers just under the skin. I have observed dramatic pain relief from both of these scar release techniques. I strongly encourage you to explore these areas further if you have had surgeries in the areas where you have pain. There are particularly good results when I inject knee scars or any scar that crosses a joint, as well as scars on the chest, abdomen, back and neck. Typically, scar injections are performed three times over the course of several weeks.

Osteopathic manipulation is a treatment mainstay in my office, as I always strive to optimize the physical structure and function of the body first. While I am an M.D., I realized early in my career how important it was to understand body mechanics. I sought out specialized training to learn osteopathic manipulative techniques at the Michigan State College of Osteopathic Medicine with the late Dr. Phil Greenman. I use this methodology with every patient I see. I strongly encourage pain management physicians to consider incorporating these techniques into their assessment and treatment of patients because it helps resolve mechanical issues quickly so that pain doesn't linger.

Chiropractic treatment varies widely based on the training of the particular doctor. There are a growing number of chiropractors who are embracing more comprehensive approaches to treating pain, not just performing weekly manipulations. I know chiropractors trained in Active Release Therapy (ART), PRI, and Functional medicine. Clearly, the more tools a practitioner has in their toolbox, the more people they can help. So, find a health-care provider who meets your needs. One of the issues we have in healthcare today is that referral systems are inefficient and it can take several weeks to get a patient into a pain specialist. I applaud chiropractors for being able to see and treat patients quickly, helping them to feel better, and move forward with their lives. Good chiropractors also know their limits and don't hesi-tate to refer patients to other doctors when more comprehensive care is needed.

TENS (transcutaneous electrical stimulation) and various forms of electrical stimulation such as microcurrent, H wave, and others of its kind have their place in the arsenal of thera-pies as well. Some are even available as home units. When your pain flares up, these modalities can be helpful 'feel good' tools.

Of course, there are other therapies and techniques that can help with pain. Some people are less open than others to explor-ing some of the less 'conventional' options. However, in the quest for relief from pain, if the 'traditional' treatments aren't helping to your satisfaction, you have nothing to lose by 'look-ing outside the box.' Of course, some of these options have ex-tensive scientific research supporting their effectiveness, such as acupuncture and massage, while others are more reliant on generations of anecdotal evidence, such as reiki, energy heal-ing, and so on.

Some examples of alternative pain therapies include:

- Acupuncture
- Naturopathy/homeopathy

- Reiki and other energy healing modalities
- Massage and manipulation
- Reflexology
- Heat and cold therapy
- Relaxation techniques - body scan meditation
- Meditation
- Visual imagery
- Breathwork
- Biofeedback
- Hypnotherapy
- Yoga, Qi Gong, and Tai Chi

Talk Therapy and the Treatment of Pain

Cognitive-Behavioral Therapy (CBT) teaches you how to have a better understanding of the real cause of your pain, helping you identify what you can do differently to improve or resolve your pain. In CBT, with the guidance of a therapist, you explore the role that pain plays in your life and what it means to you. This approach gives you a sense of control over your symptoms, making your responses to the pain more conscious and less reactive.

Acceptance and Commitment Therapy (ACT) focuses on three areas:

- Accepting your reactions and being 'present' to what is.
- Choosing a values-based direction.
- Taking action.

ACT helps you to accept the difficulties that happen in life. It's a mindfulness-based program that focuses on overcoming negative thoughts and feelings. It's values-based, which means that the therapist helps you to ensure that your values and behavior are aligned. This is important, because you can prevent distressing thoughts or avoidant behaviors that might result in negative emotions, triggering the threat response.

Another important modality is Compassion Focused Therapy (CFT), developed by Dr. Paul Gilbert, which was discussed in Chapter 2.

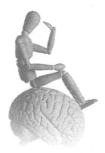

Chapter 8

Health as a Habit

"If someone wishes for good health, one must first ask oneself
if he or she is ready to do away with the reasons for their
illness. Only then is it possible to help."

- Hippocrates

I'd like to share some personal anecdotes about the importance of routines, rituals, and habits. For many decades, I used to enjoy traditional family dinners every Friday night. Around the Sabbath dinner table were four generations of my immediate family. At the beginning of every meal, my father would make a toast to everyone's good health. He would always say, 'If you have your health, then you have everything, and you can do anything.' Back then, I wondered if he might find something more topical or creative to say, but he always stuck to his routine.

With age, I have witnessed the ravages of poor health on those I love. I now recognize why my father was committed to the ritual of making that same toast at every Sabbath meal. When he was 59 years old, my father was diagnosed with lung cancer. With the diagnosis in hand, he consulted doctors locally, and then sought second and third opinions at the Memorial Sloan Kettering Cancer Center in New York and the MD Anderson Cancer Center at the University of Texas. In both instances, he was instructed to go home and get his affairs in order. This dreadful prognosis had a profound effect on our family. I remember we were all sitting on edge, waiting for that fateful day to come. Weeks went by, then months, and then years. Today, he's a vibrant 87-year-old who practices yoga or goes to the gym every day. He maintains an organic garden as well as a koi pond. He has a loving and supportive relationship with a gracious and beautiful woman. I'm blessed to have such a wonderful and supportive role model as my father, who exhibits the importance of healthy routines and daily habits.

Leading a healthy lifestyle is the product of a series of habits that requires daily discipline. Life happens, events derail our progress, and we can't fall into the trap.

I share this small part of my story with you because it's so important for us to recognize how much we are influenced by the people around us: our family, neighbors, and coworkers. When they have poor health habits, it's easy to fall into temptation and eat that donut, drink that soda, or skip the day's gym workout. When you are in a rhythm of keeping up your routines, it's usually easy to maintain. Unfortunately, healthy habits are breakable. The good news is that so are the bad habits.

When you're ready to make important changes, it's critically important to create awareness and garner the support of the people in your life. The key is that while you're ready to make the changes, the time may not be right, or your support system may not be ready to facilitate your transformation, or there may other factors standing in your way. It is helpful to have a healthy dose of realism in assessing this, as people can certainly block our progress, leading to more stress.

Some theorize that people unconsciously choose their experiences by way of the neural circuits laid down in the brain from past habits and conditioning. This same conditioning in the nervous system determines how we act physically and emotionally. Outsmarting your pain requires that you are aware of your habitual responses. Habits are a comfortable groove, but they can also be unhealthy and limiting. Healthy habits could be loosely defined as anything that soothes you, calms your nervous system, improves your mental clarity, and allows you to maintain homeostasis.

Habit Formation

Habit formation and habit change are difficult, because of the brain's set-up. According to Gardner, Lally, and Wardle, writing in the British Journal of General Practice, habits are "actions that are triggered automatically in response to contextual cues that have been associated with their performance." Most people get comfortable in their old ways. They are cued to the same responses and they make rationalizations in order to resist change. It starts with the willingness to take control over yourself.

Habit formation occurs in four stages: (adapted from National Institute of Diabetes and Digestive and Kidney Diseases)

- Contemplation - 'I am thinking about creating a new routine, but I'm not sure how I will overcome the roadblocks.' The answer lies in outlining the pros and cons of making the change.
- Preparation - 'I've made up my mind to take action.' Put goals in place and develop cues to keep yourself on track.
- Action - 'I have started to make changes.' Track your progress and reward yourself for sticking to it.

155

- Maintenance - 'I have a new routine. If I slip up every now and then, I get right back to it!'

Habit Loops

As you learned in earlier Chapters, every habit you have, both good and bad, has a habit loop. It is important to understand what the three-part loop involves.

- Cue or trigger
- Routine or behavior
- Reward

To change behaviors, you can sketch out your personal habit loop and see what you find. It might surprise you. As a reminder, here is how the habit loop works.

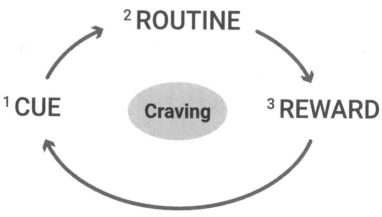

THE HABIT LOOP

² ROUTINE

¹ CUE   Craving   ³ REWARD

Adapted from Charles Duhigg

Health Habit Script

Many of us are visually-oriented. Putting our ideas on paper helps us get them out of our heads and clarify our understanding. Here's a sample script from the British Journal of General Practice. At the top of a piece of paper, write 'Make a Healthy Habit!' Then follow the steps:

- Decide on a goal that you want to achieve for your health (eat more green vegetables or get seven hours of sleep each night). So, name your goal!
- Choose a simple action that will get you towards your goal, which you can commit to doing on a daily basis.
- Plan for when and where you will do your chosen action. Choose a time and place this is consistent every day of every week. (Cue)
- Every time you encounter that time and place, do the action step. (Routine)
- It will get easier with time. Within ten weeks, you should find you're doing it automatically, without even thinking about it.
- Congratulations! You made a healthy habit! (Reward)
- Keep your sheets so you can track your progress.

In the previous chapters, I presented you with many options for improving your health by reducing the stress/threat response. I have also reminded you that there is a science to changing your health habits for the better. Knowing the science of why you do what you do will hopefully inspire you to take action steps to improve your health on all levels. As the Buddha said, "Pain is inevitable, but suffering is optional." Now you know how to opt out of suffering and outsmart your pain!

"Keep looking up! Learn from the past, dream about the future, and look up [make it a habit]. There's nothing like a beautiful sunset to end a healthy day."

- Rachel Boston

Healthy Exercise Habits

Getting Unstuck and Moving Past Pain

One of the common patterns that I see in people who make an effort to exercise is that they usually repeat the same workout every time they go to the gym. This routine creates its own set of issues by reinforcing muscle imbalances and compensatory muscle firing patterns in the body. This can lead to strain and the overuse of specific tendons. It can also lead to premature breakdown of our joints. This is an example of a 'good habit' working against you. Additionally, our brains love to learn new things, including new types of physical activity. Challenging ourselves to learn new and fun exercises and movement patterns prompts our brains to form new neural connections, helping our brains stay young, and working to mitigate the normal aging process.

In order to best deal with gravity, we need to be optimally balanced front-to-back and side-to-side. People fail to realize that our bodies are, by design, slightly asymmetrical. In addition, we live in a right hand dominant world, which impacts how we use our muscles and influences the alignment of our joints. Postural Restoration (PRI), which I have referenced previously in the book, is a physical therapy technique that recognizes these imbalances and helps restore optimal balance right-to-left and front-to-back. PRI also looks at everything from our feet on the ground, to how we stand, to how we breathe and use our core.

158

In my practice, when people get stuck, and they have a difficult time tolerating exercise, PRI therapy can be very helpful in unlocking the door to relief. PRI helps people identify what is really happening in their body. Then, they become more conscious of changes that they need to make to reduce the strain that is the result of their compensatory patterns, allowing them to optimize physical function and improve exercise tolerance.

These strategies may take people out of their comfort zone, because they become habituated to their workout routine and often resist changing it. I am amazed how people react when a health professional suggests that they change things up. The truth is that when people have poor muscle balance, their core is weak, and their breathing patterns are off-kilter, it is difficult to exercise without pain.

HITT is a Big Hit!

Exercise science is showing that thirty-minute high-intensity interval training (HIIT) workouts are the most efficient way to improve fitness. What's interesting about HIIT is that the workouts are designed to repeat bouts of significant effort, followed by brief periods of rest. The duration of the interval can be customized based on your level of fitness. Current studies show that, as compared to conventional treadmill or elliptical workouts, HIIT programs improve heart muscle function, improve oxygen consumption, improve fat burning, increase mitochondrial size, and strengthen mitochondrial function, allowing us to make more energy to fuel our lives.

The mighty mitochondria are the microscopic energy-producing structures that make up your muscles, organs, spinal cord, and brain. They use the nutrients in our food and mix it with the oxygen we breathe, processing them to generate energy for the body to function. This gives us our 'get up and go' and gives us the ability to contend with the effects of gravity. As we age, lack good nutrition, fail to get enough sleep or oxygen, or take certain types of prescription medications, our mitochondria can become impaired, reducing our energy levels, making it harder to live life to the fullest.

Other exercise approaches that are becoming more popular are methods that monitor your heart rate during sixty minute high intensity interval training sessions. This kind of non-invasive monitoring is a helpful tool to improve fitness by documenting changes over time and helping you learn where your heart rate response is at any point in time. The awareness of one's heart rate response to exercise is especially helpful for those who are just starting out and those with poor body awareness. It can also be beneficial for those seeking the ultimate challenge of what is called 'afterburn,' or excess post-exercise oxygen consumption, which helps to burn fat! One word of caution- be careful not to allow your competitive nature to take over so that you push your-self too far.

Getting to the Core of It!

In addition to HIIT, I strongly encourage people to learn about their core, which includes the respiratory diaphragm (which is a muscle), the pelvic floor muscles, and everything in between. Familiarize yourself with these critical muscles. You can find simple exercises online to start activating your core that you can do lying down on the floor in your home. You can also do simple kegel exercises to strengthen your pelvic floor. This applies to both men and women.

Your core muscles are the key to managing life's daily challenges, including both physical and emotional stressors. Your core is intimately linked with your breath and your posture, which in turn influence your autonomic nervous system function and stress/threat response. Optimizing your core muscle function and improving your breathing patterns will help you to move into a more desirable stress-resilient or parasympathetic-dominant state.

When you do not stand up straight you have more of a flexion bias (forward-stooped posture), you tend to over-strengthen your front muscles (they get tighter), as compared to your back muscles. This pattern tends to pull you forward, which impairs your balance, disrupts your breathing and circulation, makes you injury-prone, and activates your sympathetic nervous system (SNS).

Benefits of Yoga

Yoga is also a marvelous way to improve muscle balance and body awareness as a whole. Some forms of yoga focus mainly on the physical benefits, while others are beneficial for both physical and mental strength. In my recovery, I tried many different forms of yoga. One particular form of yoga that I found helpful was Kundalini Yoga, which is different in that it has a more spiritual aspect. I discovered that when your patterns of thought and behavior are particularly resistant to change, and you are stuck in self-limiting patterns, Kundalini Yoga can help you clear away old patterns that keep getting in your way.

What's most interesting about this is that they teach that by chanting specific mantras (Sanskrit prayers) and using specific hand and body postures (mudras), you can 'hack' your autonomic nervous system. This effectively calms the stress/threat response and re-establishes homeostasis giving you mastery over your nervous system, mind and emotions. Singing has a similar effect as chanting, because it also activates your recurrent laryngeal nerve, which communicates between your vocal cords and the vagus nerve.

I recommend a form of Kundalini Yoga, called Naam Yoga, developed and taught by Dr. Michael Levry who was a student and protege of spiritual teacher Yogi Bhajan. One of Dr. Levry's spiritual concepts that I find interesting is the idea that "God sits at the tip of our tongue." This could explain why our words have so much power over our reality. Dr. Levry has written many books about healing on a spiritual level and he has a worldwide following of people devoted to his teachings. Regardless of your religious orientation, or lack thereof, the potential implications of what various forms of yoga as well as these spiritual teachings have to share with us are interesting to consider.

In the course of exploring some of his teachings, I was surprised how much neuroscience was involved. I certainly gained a greater understanding of the nature and power of the autonomic nervous system as the central link in the mind-body connection. This wisdom and perspective was a valuable addition to what I learned in medical school. The saying goes that "when the student is ready, the teacher appears." Learning these teachings strongly influenced me both personally and professionally. It changed my life and I hope that it can help you as well.

All forms of yoga can help you learn specific ways of managing your stress response by teaching you to consciously manage your autonomic nervous system and improve your posture using the tools of breathing, poses, chanting, and meditation. Try different forms of yoga to find the type that is best suited for your unique needs. Some people associate yoga with meditation, but they are different. In the next section I will introduce you to a simple method of meditation called the 'body scan.'

The Body Scan Meditation

The body scan meditation is a core teaching in most mindfulness-based stress reduction (MBSR) educational programs. Unlike other types of meditation, the body scan brings awareness to the body, rather than the mind, so that you can feel or sense the effects of stress, worry, and anxiety in the body. It is recommended that you perform this practice lying down in a relaxing and supportive environment. The mediation begins with instructions to feel your left foot and then the sequence progressively draws your attention to the felt sensations in all parts of your body all the way to the top of your head.

In the process of focusing your awareness to bodily sensations, you may notice a wide range of physical feelings: pain, aches, stiffness, tingling, itches, coldness, warmth, heaviness, and more. Some of these sensations may be accompanied by thoughts or emotions. Because the body expresses what words cannot, it has its own wisdom. Learning to listen to and investigate these physical sensations, thoughts, and emotions is called the "triangle of awareness."

As you begin to enter the world of full awareness, referred to as 'being' rather than 'doing,' you may notice the impact of the feelings you have been carrying around with you that weigh you down. Here you can use RAIN to lean into unpleasant experiences and observe and allow yourself to 'be there,' without any critical thinking or judgement. You can use your breath to gently shift your focus when needed. Then you can release the emotion and the bodily sensations that accompany it.

Mindfulness can be such a helpful tool in overcoming pain. I often suggest to my patients that they practice the body scan meditation several times each week. I refer them to free and easily acces-

163

sible online resources. There are a growing number of mindfulness apps for your cell phones and tablets that host guided body scan meditations narrated by different teachers. These guided meditations are audio only. The specific sequence of focused attention you will follow during the mediation is spoken to you by the teacher. All that you need to do is lay there, listen, and feel what happens.

One meditation that I recommend to my patients is Elisha Goldstein's Body Scan Meditations hosted on *The Insight Timer* app. He offers both a 21 minute and 30 minute version. Depending on your availability of free time, you should be able to accommodate this practice into your daily routine. Mindfulness is like a muscle that needs to be exercised to get stronger. It is a sure way to fend off unnecessary pain and suffering and helps you find links between your emotions and physical sensations.

Sequencing Your Exercises

Regardless of how you like to exercise, there is a recommended sequence of introducing specific exercises at the optimal time to capitalize on the beneficial effects of neural plasticity and motor development. This is based on the notion of the neurodevelopmental sequence of crawling before you walk. Our motor patterns are, by design, somewhat hierarchical. Making sure you have the foundations laid down for walking, before running, is very important in injury prevention.

You don't want to reinforce faulty patterns. This starts with an awareness of your core and posture. Improving your balance is also key to preventing injuries. We must be stable on level surfaces before introducing unstable surfaces, such as walking on the beach or balancing on a Bosu ball. By ensuring that we're adequately balanced, and we have a normal gait, we have the foundations to be able to play sports like golf, tennis, and skiing without the fear or concern of getting injured.

Healthy Sleep Habits

Sleep is a vital part of your body's repair mechanism. When your sleep patterns are healthy, you recharge your energy for the next day, rebuild and repair tissue, and allow your digestive system to take a break. The Centers for Disease Control and Prevention (CDC) cite that 40 million Americans suffer from long-term sleep disorders and 20 million suffer from occasional sleep problems. There are many important considerations around sleep. One of the first priorities for effective sleep habits is to avoid drinking caffeinated drinks, especially after 2pm, because caffeine is a stimulant that can interfere with your circadian rhythm and disrupt your sleep.

Your Sleep Environment

Environmental factors such as an old, uncomfortable bed, as well as noise and light exposure in your bedroom, can affect your sleep. Getting a new mattress every 8 years is usually warranted, as that is the typical life expectancy of most commercially available mattresses.

If your partner or spouse has a sleep disorder, or snores loudly, this could be affecting your sleep patterns. Using sleep aids such as ear plugs would be beneficial in that circumstance. Excessive light in the bedroom is also problematic. Eye masks and blackout shades can be helpful. It is important not to be excessively exposed to 'blue light' at night from cell phones, tablets, e-readers, television, computers, and alarm clocks, as this will trigger the release of hormones in the brain that influence the natural circadian rhythm.

Another form of 'pollution,' similar to that of noise and light, applies to exposure to excessive electromagnetic radiation (EMF) from wireless routers (WiFi) and all of the computers, tablets, and cell phones that we connect to it. EMF exposure during sleep can affect your energy field, influence your heart rate and rhythm, and potentially affect your brain waves. Limiting EMF devices in the bedroom is a best practice. At a minimum, I would recommend unplugging your WiFi during the sleeping hours.

All of the technological advancements that we enjoy, while important for relaxation in the evenings, reduce production of melatonin, which is critical for helping us to go to sleep. If possible, avoid the use of electronic devices, or looking at screens, in the hour or two prior to bedtime. Alternatively, you can purchase inexpensive blue-light blocking glasses. It would also be helpful to keep all of these kinds of electronic devices out of your bedroom, so as to avoid temptation, with the added benefit of reducing EMF exposure.

Another problem with electronic usage before bed is that, whether or not we realize it, exposure to the news media, with all of its drama and hysteria, can have dramatic effects on our stress response mechanism. Limiting your exposure in the hours before bedtime will help you sleep better.

Learning to Shut off Your Mind

Many people tell me that they simply cannot 'shut off' their mind at night, causing them to lose out on sleep. Mental over-stimulation is a huge source of stress. Following the above steps to address environmental conditions and limit media exposure at night will be very helpful in improving your sleep.

Also, learning specific techniques to quiet the mind through conscious breathing techniques is also very beneficial. I routinely teach my patients the 'Relaxing Breath' method, also called the 4-7-8 breathing pattern, which has been popularized by Dr. Andrew Weil. Because of the beneficial effects of conscious breath regulation on our nervous system, Dr. Weil asserts that this technique "acts like a natural tranquilizer for the nervous system." There are other physiologic benefits of this type of breathing, including removing carbon dioxide (CO_2) and optimizing our body's pH level. This impacts pain and inflammation, because when we retain CO_2, and our pH is lower (more acidic), we tend to be in a pro-inflammatory state. When we expel CO_2, our pH increases, becoming more alkaline. This makes us less susceptible to the effects of inflammation.

4-7-8 Breathing

This is a simple way to help you get to sleep. Dr. Weil has a short YouTube video on this technique, but the basic steps are as follows:

- Exhale completely through your mouth, making a low-level whooshing sound.
- Close your mouth and inhale quietly through your nose to a mental count of four.
- Hold your breath for a count of seven.
- Exhale completely through your mouth, making the whooshing sound to a count of eight. (This is the most important step in relaxing the body)
- Repeat the cycle three more times for a total of four breaths.

CBD Oil

A relatively new option for the treatment of pain is CBD oil, which is an effective and naturally occurring painkiller. It is a phytocannabinoid, meaning that it is the non-psychoactive part of the cannabis plant. Cannabidiol oil is an extract of the hemp plant, which makes it different than marijuana in that hemp has less than 0.3 percent THC and marijuana has greater amounts.

Studies show that one of the chief effects of CBD oil is reducing inflammation, which can alleviate pain. It may also help with neuropathic or nerve pain working through centrally mediated pain mechanisms. CBD oil has been shown to be a 'neuromodulator' for several physiological processes that keep us alive and healthy. It may be helpful in the treatment of Fibromyalgia and Multiple Sclerosis (MS). Unlike opioids, CBD oil reportedly does not lose its effectiveness over time.

I should be clear that some of the studies on CBD oil have not been evaluated by the Food and Drug Administration (FDA) and there is some controversy surrounding the many uses of this product. While the risk of 'overdose' is low, and the side effects seem quite mild, you need to be the best judge as to what is best for you.

If you choose to try CBD oil, I suggest that you start with a low dose and titrate the dosage slowly so that you see a clear effect. Most importantly, make sure you don't make it a habit. There are currently no genuine standards for gauging the actual 'potency' of the CBD oil that is currently available in health food stores as well as online. The question as to whether it is legal in various states is also somewhat controversial. I suggest you research the laws that apply to your state so as to avoid any unnecessary controversy or legal difficulty.

While I am not an expert in the use of CBD oil, the available scientific literature shows that, when used as a dietary supplement, it may have the following potential benefits:

- May protect brain cells and helps with neuro-regeneration.
- May reverse cognitive decline from Alzheimer's disease.
- May quell anxiety and help with PTSD and stress.

- May help with depression.
- May help with sleep.

Medication for Sleep

When we have trouble sleeping, we first need to figure out why. Our ability to sleep is extremely sensitive to stress and worry. We should consider sleep issues as an early warning sign that the effects of stress are starting to build up. Ironically, sleepless nights cause people to get increasingly worried and stressed, which is why they start enlisting the aid of sleeping pills.

The CDC reports that nine million Americans use prescription sleeping drugs, and the numbers are continuing to rise. Psychiatrist Allen Frances asserts, "sleeping pills are so massively overutilized in part because there is no accepted gold standard of normal sleep. Individual variation is great in the number of hours needed, timing of falling asleep and waking up, and how refreshed people feel in the morning."

However, proactively preventing insomnia is much wiser than taking medication to facilitate sleep. When simple solutions will work for sleep dysfunction, it is not prudent to take sleeping pills. Many of these pharmaceutical sleep aids are simply ineffective, or worse, can become 'habit forming' for the same reasons as opioids.

It is reported that as many as 40 percent of insomniacs do not respond to sleeping pills. Most guidelines about the proper use of sleeping pills dictate that they should be used for short-term use only (four weeks maximum). The elderly are particularly vulnerable to the negative effects of sleeping pills, because they tend to become easily disoriented, have a higher risk of falls, and they don't easily metabolize the drugs.

Because of the controversies surrounding the long-term use of prescription sleep aids, new resources for sleep are available, including Sleepio.com. This is an online sleep improvement program that employs cognitive behavioral approaches.

Healthy Nutrition Habits

Cliché as it may be, it is absolutely, albeit metaphorically, true that 'we are what we eat.' The foods we eat are either good medicine or toxins. In fact, the best preventative medicine that doctors can prescribe includes proper nutrition and adequate hydration. Eating well means eating a balance of proteins, carbohydrates, and fats. It also required that we get adequate vitamins, minerals, and water. The human body is between 60 to 70 percent water and optimal daily water intake is eight to ten glasses of clean water daily.

The reality is that dehydration is the most easily preventable medical condition in the world. It has been reported that 75 percent of Americans are chronically dehydrated. This is partly because caffeinated drinks actually dehydrate us, contributing to the problem. Many people advocate filtering your water to remove excess chlorine, chloramines, and fluoride. These chemicals are added into our water supply to maintain 'water quality,' though there is a debate about how much they benefit us. Some people argue that these chemicals, especially fluoride, are toxic to the body and brain. Drinking alkaline water with a pH of 8 to 9 is also controversial, but some people believe that the alkalinity helps to reduce inflammation in the body, potentially reversing some of the harmful effects of our modern lifestyles.

Avoiding foods that are genetically modified and highly processed is also important for our health. I also suggest eliminating artificial sweeteners and other food additives such as MSG that our bodies are not equipped to handle. There are many resources out there oriented specifically towards healthy nutrition. I suggest the Whole30 Program for comprehensive diet and nutrition education about healthy eating habits. For people with irritable bowel syndrome, I recommend a food elimination diet to see what foods are triggering your 'leaky gut.' The four most common culprits for food intolerance leading to leaky gut are gluten, dairy, eggs, and peanuts. After that, I suggest you look at how soy and corn affects you.

For those people with arthritis, I recommend limiting intake of nightshade vegetables and considering a food elimination diet starting with some of the foods listed above. Much less common are issues with foods that are high in oxalates and lectins. These two food groups are tricky because they appear to be what we would generally consider high in phytonutrients (plant-based nutrition). In reality, it is believed that, for some people, these foods actually prevent the absorption of other beneficial nutrients, because they chelate or bind to various minerals, preventing absorption.

Lectins are found in legumes, such as string beans and grains. Foods high in oxalates include dark chocolate, nuts, berries, citrus fruits, kale, spinach, zucchini, beets, and sweet potatoes. People with a history of kidney stones and irritable bowel syndrome (IBS) might consider limiting these foods. Since these foods are hard to avoid, it is best to limit quantities in our daily diet. For those who like green smoothies to boost their nutrition, low oxalate green powders are available.

Healthy Dietary Supplements

Prudent use of nutritional supplements is advised. People who are healthy, eat good food, and drink adequate amounts of clean water usually still require some nutritional supplementation. However, the longer one goes on eating poorly, drinking alcohol or caffeine excessively, sleeping poorly, and suffering the ill effects of stress, the greater the level of supplementation that may be needed.

Beyond the limited recommendation of essential nutritional support supplements, elaborating on the wide range of nutraceuticals is beyond the scope of this book. I do recommend that everyone have their vitamin D2 levels checked annually, as this critical nutrient is essential to our musculoskeletal and immune system function. Most laboratories cite the normal range as 32 to 100, but I assert that these ranges are arbitrary. In my experience, optimal health is best achieved when the Vitamin D2 level is in an ideal range of 60 to 80.

Vitamin D is available in two forms. Vitamin D2 is the inactive form, while Vitamin D3 is the active form. When we ingest food containing Vitamin D, we absorb D2, and the sun then converts D2 into the active form D3. When Vitamin D levels are low, optimal supplementation would consist of a combination of the prescription Vitamin D2 (50,000 IU taken weekly) and Vitamin D3 taken daily (ranging from 1,000 to 5,000 IU).

I also recommend magnesium supplementation to many of my patients, provided that they have normal kidney function. Magnesium is helpful in many respects, as it helps absorb Vitamin D, and works to prevent headaches and muscle cramps.

CoQ10 is another helpful nutraceutical that improves mitochondrial function. It also works to counter the negative effects of cholesterol-lowering statin drugs.

A comprehensive multi-vitamin/multi-mineral, coupled with a high-potency Vitamin B complex, are also important for optimizing our mitochondrial energy production and supporting overall health. For those who drink alcohol regularly, ask your doctor to check your Vitamin B12 and folic acid levels, and supplement with extra Vitamin B6. I also recommend Vitamin C supplementation for its antioxidant effects (2,000mg daily), as well as fish oil and turmeric (curcumin) as natural anti-inflammatory agents. Probiotics are also helpful in maintaining a healthy gut microbiome.

Healthy Habit Takeaways

Concerning the value of healthy habits, Anne Wilson Schaef asserts that, "Good health is not something we can buy. However, it can be an extremely valuable savings account." I believe this is in keeping with Benjamin Franklin's adage that "an ounce of prevention is worth a pound of cure." The bottom line is to take care of your health and make it your greatest asset.

Generally speaking, when creating healthy habits, I suggest the following action items:

- Practice your habits early in the morning, when you are fresh, and your willpower is at its peak.
- Set small achievable goals and actions that matter.
- Be prepared with everything you need. Pack your lunch, snacks, and enough pure water to help you get through the day. This way you will be less tempted to consume unhealthy foods on the fly.
- Make it fun and convenient.
- Find a tribe of people with similar values and goals.
- Try not to break the chain. It takes 66 days to form a new habit, so keep it going and chart your progress.
- Stay focused on the big picture.

- Be accountable to yourself. People with step trackers and fitness monitors walk 27 percent more than those who don't.
- Forgive yourself if you slip up, and then move on.
- Look at each morning as a new opportunity.

"The difference between try and triumph is just a little umph."

- Anonymous

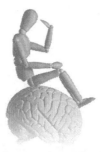

Chapter 9

Pain Metaphors

"The body is but a vessel for the soul."

- A.J. Durai

Your body is the physical manifestation of your pain and your joy. You literally carry your stress in every cell and tissue of your body, because you are always responding though your psychoneuroimmunology to the state of your heart and mind. This is why, when you are under times of stress and despair, you have trouble breathing, thinking straight, experience heart palpitations, and have that queasy feeling in your stomach.

It's hard to deny that emotional pain isn't felt as physical discomfort and that joy is felt as a sense of lightness and calm. It has everything to do with which neurotransmitters are being released by the brain in each moment. Remember that when your brain releases serotonin, dopamine, or oxytocin your body feels good and you are happy. On the other hand, when you feel threatened, stress kicks in, cortisol and adrenaline are released, and you experience sensations of dread. This is when we slip into survival mode.

We all have situations in our lives that are less than ideal. Sometimes they are centered around our internal 'demons', while at other times, the demons belong to those with whom we live and work and even prior generations of our family. Awareness of the huge impact these factors have on your suffering, or health, is essential. Learning to delve into all of the parts of your life that contribute to your pain is essential to healing.

Healthy habits aren't just limited to eating well, exercising regularly, and sleeping seven to eight hours a night. Developing true healthy habits requires you to do an objective appraisal of yourself. This evaluation starts internally. For starters, ask yourself some important questions. How do you think and feel emotionally? What's driving you? What's making you unhappy? What brings you joy? What makes you feel good and brings a sense of peace and calm? The next step is to clear out the physical clutter and take stock of the toxic elements in your life, which keep you fixed and prevent you from making positive changes.

Holding onto things, people, and situations is part of everyone's nature. Change is hard, but holding on becomes a habit. At a certain point, the burden of carrying all of this stuff around with you becomes too heavy. Your health starts to suffer, because the demands exceed your carrying capacity for stress. Things can get so piled up that it's hard to see the one thing you can do that might have the biggest impact.

In my experience, even when you recognize the things in your life that are out of balance, the power of fear may make you hesitant to take action. Sometimes we even fear the notion of being successful, so we self-sabotage just when we should be moving forward and taking positive action. Remember that faulty beliefs, and the resulting cascade of physiological effects, are often left over from past experiences and are filtered out of our current

176

point of view. Pushback from other people's defensiveness and resistance to our desired change, as well as their desire to impose their will on us, can also trigger our stress/threat response.

Pain Metaphors

Metaphors are described by George Lakoff and Mark Johnson as "a way of conceiving of one thing in terms of another, and its primary function is to gain understanding." Understanding pain is difficult and languaging pain has its challenges by virtue of our conditioning to resist it. Nonetheless, metaphors can help us find the thread of meaning and understanding that our pain has to share with us, without triggering unnecessary anxiety, fear, and stress.

I have a patient who doesn't smoke, yet during every appointment, he comes to my office smelling of cigarette smoke. When he first came to see me, he was experiencing severe neck pain. He was on multiple medications and had frequent headaches. He explained to me that he lives in a beautiful, historic home on a river just off of the Chesapeake Bay, with the most amazing coastal views. His wife lives in the house with him, and unfortunately, she smokes incessantly. He revealed that they sleep in separate bedrooms and don't have much in the way of positive interactions. When I first saw him, I theorized that, this was a great metaphor- although his house appears outwardly beautiful, it's actually a deeply toxic environment.

On the outside, his house and property were stunning, like something out of the Architectural Digest or Town & Country. But on the inside, it was a total health hazard. He couldn't see what was happening because he was used to living in those conditions. When it became clear, after a couple of visits, that he had no intention of leaving that environment and believed he was

177

powerless to change it, we started to brainstorm small changes he could make to improve his overall health. Receiving information from, and being affected by our environment, is entirely human, and is important to every level of our health and wellness.

His pain metaphors were obvious, given that his chief complaints were neck pain and headaches. In the world of 'pain metaphors,' his neck symptoms could be interpreted as a block in his ability to express his true feelings about what he needs to be healthy. Alternatively, one could say that his wife is a 'pain in his neck' because she was not being supportive of his health or her own. Her all-or-nothing thinking made it difficult for him to feel supported. When he expressed to me his fear that any changes would push her buttons, I encouraged him to start small.

I knew that, unless we could start to make inroads to clean up his external and internal environments, it would be especially challenging to solve any of his pain problems. I explained to him that we could perform some cortisone injections in his neck, as well as explore the possibility of radiofrequency ablation if he responds temporarily to the diagnostic nerve blocks. However, I advised him that unless he makes some changes to his circumstances at home, I was concerned that the treatment would fail because his mental and emotional worlds were still overly stressful. In fact, he returned to my office several times, each time reporting that he experienced some limited relief from the procedures. I made additional suggestions for change, such as getting a HEPA filter to detoxify the air in his bedroom. I also encouraged him to get a new bed and start weaning himself from the old worn-out recliner chair he had been sleeping in for years. The extent to which I will be able to help him resolve his pain is an open question.

This example illustrates how our external and internal pressures come to bear on how we feel physically and emotionally.

He was clearly seeking help with pain, but his pain was only the tip of the iceberg. He had insufficient awareness of what lay beneath the surface.

Learning to listen to our own aches and pains helps us understand what our subconscious mind is trying to tell us through the metaphor of our pain. Thus, pain metaphors can be a helpful cue to find the important threads in our lives - where we carry the most stress - that need to be inspected, accepted, and then snipped. Many different models of pain maps have been developed, which reflect where certain emotions are stored in the body.

In the paragraphs below, I will explore some general theories and principles of how pain is experienced in the body. The information shared in the paragraphs below represent a composite of what I have learned from many sources over several decades of studying the mind-body connection. You will not find this information in a medical textbook. It is part of your unique pain story. Because 'our biography becomes our biology,' I offer you this information as a tool to help you better understand yourself, as well as help you identify hidden triggers that may be affecting your health. I hope you find these metaphors interesting to consider.

Pain in the lower extremities:

- Pain in the right leg slows you down from your hectic life, and metaphorically asks you to identify where you feel unsupported in your career and finances and reflects to us fear of change.
- Left leg pain can be associated with unresolved issues from the past, recalling a lack of emotional support or not feeling safe.

- The left groin area is the betrayal center reflecting back to us, when we feel betrayed by another or when we betray ourselves.
- Left hip pain can reflect a fear of moving forward.
- Right-sided groin issues are where we tend to store abandonment issues.
- Knee pain can reflect whether we are being inflexible or unforgiving with ourselves or others. Resentment can also be associated with the knees, as well as issues of surrender and devotion.
- The ankles are the centers of emotion. Swollen ankles might suggest a build-up of unexpressed emotion.

Pain in the hip and low back can suggest we have a lack of support, either emotional, financial, or both. This area of the body reflects safety and security. Consequences of our childhood can show up here as well. Our lower back is also considered our relationship sector. Do we feel supported in our relationships? If not, we need to pull on the threads of these pain metaphors to find our hidden triggers?

Pain in the areas of the abdomen and pelvis:

- Pelvic pain and pelvis issues, especially in women, can reflect fear of survival and a past history of abuse. Exploring this kind of pain metaphor in a safe therapeutic environment can be life changing.
- Pain in the right side of the belly, reflects anger at our self or others, and also implies jealousy or resentment. This can present as gall bladder issues, fatty liver, and so on.
- Pain in the left side of the belly symbolizes guilt and self-judgment. Some of us have difficulty giving and receiving. This is reflected in left-sided pain issues.

- Our stomach area corresponds to our solar plexus and is the seat of fear in the body. When we give our power away to people, things, jobs, substances, gambling, and bad habits, we feel pain and symptoms here. For example, this could manifest physically as a stomach ulcer or reflux.

Pain in the chest and neck:

- As you might imagine, pain in the heart and lung areas reflect relationships, grief, and sorrow. Sometimes a sense of helplessness, aloneness, embarrassment, and shame manifests here. This is also where we experience a lack of emotional support.
- Pain in the neck and throat area is reflective of lack of trust, fear of self-expression, and fear of abandonment or retribution. Also, a lack of forgiveness can be associated with the neck. This can be seen in throat cancer, thyroid disease, and neck pain. The neck is the bridge between our head and our heart. Things can get stuck there, which disrupts our ability to fully feel joy.
- Headaches can represent unexpressed feelings, worry, and anxiety as well as self-doubt. Headaches can also indicate resistance to life, desire to control, and disconnection from the body. Analysis paralysis comes to mind when one has headaches.

Pain in the upper extremities:

- Our right shoulder reflects the emotional burdens of carrying the weight of the world on our shoulders.
- The left shoulder is suggestive of perfectionism and holding onto internal burdens without letting them go.

- Elbow pain can symbolize a lack of flexibility and resistance to change and can involves issues of boundaries.
- Hand pain can occur when we need to reach out to others. We may have a lack of friendship and support.

Below is a composite diagram of much of what you have learned above. Interestingly, if you search this topic online, you will find many similar 'maps' of the emotional centers in your body. As such, it's hard to credit one source. For me personally, my dear friend and mentor, Dr. Cynthia Bischoff, has been a great teacher in this and many other areas. I encourage you to visit her website at www.heartliving.com for more information.

EMOTIONAL CENTERS OF THE BODY

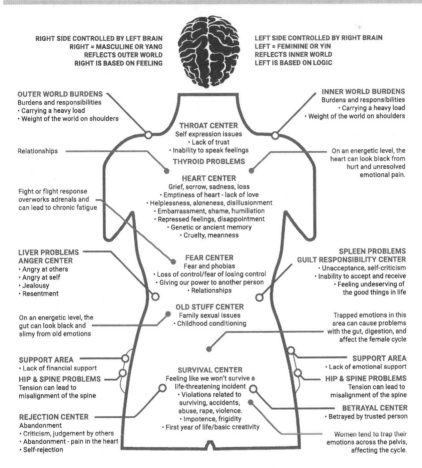

RIGHT SIDE CONTROLLED BY LEFT BRAIN
RIGHT = MASCULINE OR YANG
REFLECTS OUTER WORLD
RIGHT IS BASED ON FEELING

LEFT SIDE CONTROLLED BY RIGHT BRAIN
LEFT = FEMININE OR YIN
REFLECTS INNER WORLD
LEFT IS BASED ON LOGIC

OUTER WORLD BURDENS
Burdens and responsibilities
· Carrying a heavy load
· Weight of the world on shoulders

INNER WORLD BURDENS
Burdens and responsibilities
· Carrying a heavy load
· Weight of the world on shoulders

THROAT CENTER
Self expression issues
· Lack of trust
· Inability to speak feelings
THYROID PROBLEMS

Relationships

On an energetic level, the
heart can look black from
hurt and unresolved
emotional pain.

HEART CENTER
Grief, sorrow, sadness, loss
· Emptiness of heart - lack of love
· Helplessness, aloneness, disillusionment
· Embarrassment, shame, humiliation
· Repressed feelings, disappointment
· Genetic or ancient memory
· Cruelty, meanness

Fight or flight response
overworks adrenals and
can lead to chronic fatigue

**LIVER PROBLEMS
ANGER CENTER**
· Angry at others
· Angry at self
· Jealousy
· Resentment

FEAR CENTER
Fear and phobias
· Loss of control/fear of losing control
· Giving our power to another person
· Relationships

**SPLEEN PROBLEMS
GUILT RESPONSIBILITY CENTER**
· Unacceptance, self-criticism
· Inability to accept and receive
· Feeling undeserving of
the good things in life

On an energetic level, the
gut can look black and
slimy from old emotions

OLD STUFF CENTER
Family sexual issues
· Childhood conditioning

Trapped emotions in this
area can cause problems
with the gut, digestion, and
affect the female cycle

SUPPORT AREA
· Lack of financial support
HIP & SPINE PROBLEMS
Tension can lead to
misalignment of the spine

SURVIVAL CENTER
Feeling like we won't survive a
life-threatening incident
· Violations related to
surviving, accidents,
abuse, rape, violence.
· Impotence, frigidity
· First year of life/basic creativity

SUPPORT AREA
· Lack of emotional support
HIP & SPINE PROBLEMS
Tension can lead to
misalignment of the spine

REJECTION CENTER
Abandonment
· Criticism, judgement by others
· Abandonment - pain in the heart
· Self-rejection

BETRAYAL CENTER
· Betrayed by trusted person

Women tend to trap their
emotions across the pelvis,
affecting the cycle.

Problems with the legs/knees/ankles on the right side can reflect
feelings of lack of support in career and finances. Can also be a
signal that you need to slow down to take stock of the situation.

Problems with the legs/knees/ankles on the left side can reflect
feelings of lack of emotional support. Old injuries that still cause pain
are due to unresolved emotional stuff and can be evident for years.

Our body is a reflection of our subconscious mind, and our body speaks to us in metaphors. This is what it really means to be human and we all have to deal with it sooner or later. With these new insights, you can now identify the healthy changes you need to make in how you think and feel. This is how you heal from the inside out!

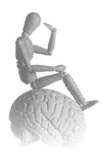

Epilogue
The Transformational Aspects of Pain

"I have found the paradox that if you love until it hurts, there can be no more hurt, only more love."

- Mother Teresa

Pain is a wake-up call! When the pain alarm sounds, your stress and threat levels are too high, and change is necessary. Remember that your body is wise and your symptoms are your teachers. Experiencing pain and suffering doesn't mean the universe is out to get you; it just means your life is out of balance and change is called for. Change is a necessity of life and resistance to change causes pain. This is a paradox we all face sooner or later. The good news is that liberation and joy are byproducts of going through change; pain is the byproduct of resisting it. This is how pain transforms us!

We are all wired for pain, but we're also equipped to be able to change the circumstances perpetuating our pain. Learning to cope with trauma and pain, without triggering your nervous system, helps you discover the path to self-mastery, growth, and healing. On our journey through life, when we face our challenges, we often experience a period of 'post-traumatic growth.' This 'down time' allows us to process and incorporate what we have learned. This is when we gain perspective.

It's an opportunity for empowerment, translating into unshakable personal strength, increased self-confidence, and growing determination. These 'heroic' traits, along with your expanding sense of healthy empathy and compassion, become the tools you will use to overcome your pain habits and be in a position to help others. The key is to face your challenges, rather than hiding from them. If you hide in denial, or resist change, the prize of unshakable peace will remain just outside your reach. Mindfulness techniques can help and studies show clear efficacy.

Learning mindfulness and mindfulness-based stress reduction techniques has been demonstrated by researchers at Carnegie Mellon University to reduce inflammatory markers in the blood. It is clear that there are biological health-related benefits associated with mindfulness practices, because they actually alter the wiring patterns in the brain. This is the power of neuroplasticity!

Functional MRI studies actually show that after an eight-week mindfulness-based stress reduction program, the brain's fight-or-flight center in the amygdala appears to shrink. According to Tom Ireland, this primal region of the brain, associated with fear and emotion, is involved in the initiation of the body's response to stress. Ireland asserts that "as the amygdala shrinks, the prefrontal cortex - associated with higher order brain functions such as awareness, concentration and decision making - becomes thicker."

Studies also show that certain qualities of extraversion, openness, and optimism help facilitate growth. They also show that your social support system, as well as your willingness to think differently (mentally pivot), help you develop the wisdom needed to transform your old 'pain story' to a new vibrant life narrative.

Pain Stories

Your experience of pain is highly influenced by the labels and judgments you attach to it. 'I have always had a bad back.' 'The pain is too much to bear.' 'I'm miserable.' These are examples of 'stories' that people tell about their pain. Whenever I hear my patients comment negatively about their pain, I challenge them to change their story.

I explain to them that words have power over the subconscious mind, which takes everything we say literally, as you learned earlier in the book. It's best not to make any negative suggestions, because it's equivalent to planting negative hypnotic suggestions into your brain for action. Like a football quarterback running the wrong play, this is the ultimate form of self-sabotage. Rather than talking your body into pain, I suggest you ask yourself small, but important questions every day to gain a better understanding of why you hurt.

Learn to recognize your personal stress/threat response patterns, so that you can become aware of the early warning signs. Recognize and acknowledge the resources you have around you that will help you find safe ways to initiate change. Rather than listing all of the things that you can't do because of the pain, contemplate the things that restore you. Write out your self-care rituals. Having a morning grounding and calming routine can help set the pace and tone of the day.

'Practicing the pause' during the course of the day also helps to reset your nervous system, preventing escalating stress responses. Check in with your posture and your breathing patterns. Many of my patients find that when they maintain a gratitude journal every night before they go to bed, they feel better. No matter how severe their pain was, they realize they still have something to feel grateful for. These techniques help to rewire your brain in positive ways, making neuroplasticity work for you, not against you.

Here's an exercise to help you to reframe and rebuild you story. Imagine you're living in the future. You decide to write a book about your experience with pain. In writing the book, you look back and think about what you learned from your challenges. From this fresh perspective, you tell the story of how pain changed your life by making you a stronger person, showing parts of yourself you had not previously recognized. You begin to contextualize your pain in a different light, recognizing its deeper meaning. This creates feelings of strength and mastery that can lead to peace and calm.

People who don't like to write stories can write affirmations, which are simple statements that go straight into the subconscious mind, helping to rewire your brain in positive ways. Here are some examples of affirmations:

- I have the power to heal.
- I am stronger than any pain I might feel.
- I trust my body.
- I embrace my body. My pain is part of me, but doesn't define me.
- The power to heal exists within me.
- Illness doesn't define me.

- I am stronger than my pain.
- I am strong and resilient in the face of life's challenges.
- I accept my life as it is.
- Faith in myself is my anchor through all my troubles.
- I control my fate and where I am is where I am supposed to be.
- I experience everything in my life for a reason, including my pain.
- My pain will stimulate my growth as a person, helping me to develop compassion, perspective, and wisdom.

These affirmations were adapted in part from www.alternativeresourcesdirectory.com.

In general, affirmations are most effective when they are highly specific to you. Ideally, they should reflect your innermost needs and not those of others. They must be believable. While I encourage you to shoot for the stars, it may be more practical to start with baby steps. Practice the process until it becomes second nature to you. Practice feeling the affirmations in your cells. Remember that the main purpose of affirmations is to reprogram beliefs that are held in your subconscious mind. This is the mind-body connection in action.

The body are made up of atoms and 60 to 70 percent water. Our atoms are in constant motion, suspended in a fluid matrix. This 'atomic soup' is in a constant state of motion. In his book *The Hidden Messages in Water,*' Dr. Masaru Emoto demonstrates how our thoughts, feelings, and emotions, as well as our environment, all impact the shape of the water molecules that constitute our unique cellular matrix. When we are in a positive state of mind, our water molecules align into beautiful crystals. When we are in a negative state of mind, and feel stressed, our crystals become disfigured. This may explain how homeostasis is a different experience in the body than distress. The implications of Dr. Emoto's work are far reaching in terms of understanding health, wellness, pain, and disease. I encourage you to consider his work as living proof of the main messages in this book.

Choose Wisely, My Friend!

Now you know the secret! Conscious choices are the key to health. Real choices stem from a place of inner freedom, rather than as fear-based reactions or automatic/ingrained response patterns. The root of true empathy and compassion lies in knowing that we are all driven by the same basic desire in life: to be happy and free from suffering! We are all capable of choosing to be happy. I am especially fond of Bill Butler's acronym 'CHOICES,' because it is solution focused.

Continually

Harnessing

Opportunities

In

Creating

Excellent

Solutions

Speaking of the topic of choices and the mind-body connection, Dr. Cynthia Bischoff, teaches that if we choose to see it this way, "pain and illness can be a tool for transformation of more than just your physical self." She also asserts that "the purpose of every illness is to help change you in some way." However, you may not realize this until you take personal responsibility for identifying the true nature of your pain or illness.

I believe that pain is the intimate private messenger that holds the answers to our healing and freedom from suffering. Just recognize and remember that pain can be your nemesis, or it can be your greatest gift. The distinction rests in your perception. Transforming something that seems terrible into something positive requires the right perspective. These are your keys to healing. I hope they empower you to ignite your own personal transformational experience!

Learn Daily Practices for Transformation:

- Love yourself; it's a survival need.
- Release negative thoughts.
- Relax fully and be in the present moment.
- Laugh for no reason.
- Move your body freely and listen to music.
- Set positive intentions and say them out loud.
- Practice the pause regularly and check-in with your body.
- Create some feel-good rituals. They will nurture you.
- Journal and ask yourself questions.
- Create a sacred space that makes you feel safe.
- Breathe consciously. It's free!
- Do nothing. Really! Take a day or an afternoon off.
- Start to inventory where your attention goes during the course of the day.
- Suspend judgment and be okay with what is.
- Ground your energy and connect with nature.
- Drink more water. Your health depends on it.

- Smile for no reason.
- Have faith in yourself.
- Be clear about and embrace your personal values.
- Set firm boundaries.
- Believe in possibility and be open to synchronicity.
- Own your power to choose.
- Suspend your disbelief and release resistance.
- Be grateful. It's contagious!
- Make self-exploration and self-healing a lifelong habit.
- Make health a habit.
- Above all, forgive yourself.
- Practice makes perfect.

"To enjoy good health, to bring true happiness to your family, to bring peace to all, you must first discipline and control your own mind. If you can control your mind, you can find the way to Enlightenment, and all wisdom and virtue will naturally come to you."

- Buddha

For helpful tools and tips to help you overcome pain
and transform your life, go to my website
www.LisaBarrMD.com

or my Facebook page
https://www.facebook.com/LisaBarrMD

Expanded resources for this book, including a references list
and an index, will be located on my website.

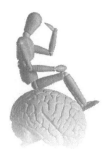

About the Author

Lisa Barr, M.D. is a #1 international bestselling author and a native of Hampton Roads, Virginia. She is a seasoned board-certified physician specializing in treating pain. She has over 30 years of medical experience. Her passion for finding unique solutions for people with painful musculoskeletal conditions has consistently garnered her recognition and acclaim.

In her clinical practice as a physiatrist (Physical Medicine and Rehabilitation), Dr. Barr focuses on innovative methods to help guide people to optimal recovery, assisting each person to achieve their best functional outcome. By embracing both the newest technologies and the 'fine art of healing,' she is recognized as a driving force of change in the medical field both locally and nationally. Over the past 20 years, she has pioneered a range of regenerative medicine modalities that facilitate the body to heal itself, including platelet-rich plasma (PRP) and stem cell therapies.

She was the first physician in coastal Virginia to integrate these techniques into her unique medical model, which also includes traditional interventional pain management, osteopathic manipulation, use of diagnostic musculoskeletal ultrasound, energy work, mind-body medicine, and Integrative and Functional medicine. Her patients range in age from teenagers to seniors and vary across a wide swathe of occupations, including professional and amateur athletes, dancers, firefighters, military personnel, boardroom executives, busy homemakers, proud grandparents, and much more.

Dr. Barr has consistently been honored by her peers as a 'Top Doc'. In 2012, she was selected as one of her region's Business Women of the Year.

As a healer, teacher and innovator at heart, Dr. Barr's mission is to promote pain literacy and empower people to harness the mind-body connection, so we can all live pain-free, become more resilient, and achieve optimal health.

Made in the USA
Columbia, SC
16 August 2019